Equine Nutrition:
From a Species Appropriate Perspective

Applied Equine Ecology Series, Vol I

Sarah L Reagan, CVND, CEqN, HD(RHom)

"Crops are the creative connection
between the soil and animal health"

William Albrecht

Equine Nutrition:
From a Species Appropriate Perspective

Sarah L Reagan, CVND, CEqN, HD(RHom)

Applied Equine Ecology Series, Vol I

USA

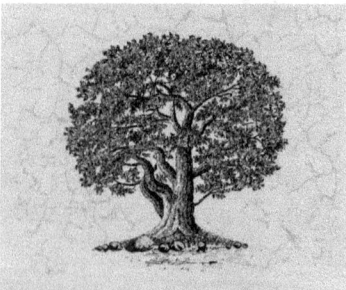

Willow Oak Publishing
Knoxville, TN USA

Dedication and Acknowledgments

This book is dedicated to *all the Horses*, and especially those who have touched my life. This is but a small attempt to repay a huge debt of gratitude for unselfish love and an education that has no rival in any brick and mortar building.

I wish to thank Drs. Kim Bloomer and Jeannie Thomason for giving me the opportunity to use the American Council of Animal Naturopathy's online education platform as an outlet for me to do what I love best – write and teach others about the nature of horses.

Photo, diagram, and table credit sources are listed with each placement. If the source is unknown, it is listed as such. Shutterstock photos are allowed under a limited license for up to 250,000 copies (http://www.shutterstock.com/licensing.mhtml).

CONTENTS

TABLE OF FIGURES

PREFACE

This publication is the first of an anticipated series collectively designated as the *Applied Equine Ecology Series*. This book was initially conceived as a certification course to be delivered by the American Council of Animal Naturopathy (www.animalnaturopathy.org), and is thus primarily structured as a text. However the necessity of making this and upcoming publications available to readers not desiring certification became apparent, and so is being published in the marketplace for anyone interested in the information contained herein.

If you are interested in certification, please contact the American Council of Animal Naturopathy at info@animalnaturopathy.org or (505) 221-6108 during the hours of 8:00 AM - 4:00 PM Pacific Time (11:-00 AM - 7:00 PM Eastern Time). A.C.A.N. is the only organization in North America to date that offers certification courses and continuing education in both small animal and equine naturopathy. A.C.A.N. was founded in March 2011 by Kim Bloomer, CVND and Jeanette (Jeannie) Thomason, CVND.

Disclaimer

I have made every effort towards the goal of accuracy in researching and writing this book. I, nor anyone associated with this book in any way, including the American Council of Animal Naturopathy and its board members, take responsibility for any results – positive or negative – that may occur from reliance on the information contained within this book. When one is dealing with a living, breathing animal, there are dynamics that come into play that cannot logically be covered in any one publication. Thus, the information provided here is for educational purposes and it is the ultimate responsibility of the owner/caretaker to make any decisions regarding the care – nutritional or otherwise – of the horse. Horses are large animals and as such, any associated activities carry a certain amount of risk, which is the sole responsibility of the person charged with the care of the horse.

I am not a licensed veterinarian and in no way attempt to represent myself as such. Nothing in this book should be construed as diagnosis, treatment, or veterinary advice as is currently defined by the American Veterinary Medical Association or any other local, regional, or national body that has the authority to promulgate veterinary medical definitions.

I

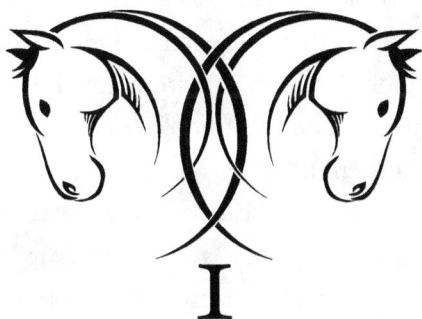

INTRODUCTION

I SUPPOSE IT WOULD be best to tell you first what this book is not about. This is not another book just about NRC (National Research Council) feeding recommendations for your horse; they are easily found. It is not about which concentrated or compound feed is the best for your horse. It is not about how to micromanage your horse's dietary intake for whatever "use" he is put to. It is, however, a perspective on how to feed your horse that reaches outside the current norms; a perspective that is grounded in the laws of nature and that is based upon the physiological requirements of the species. It is a multidisciplinary perspective that not only recognizes the laboratory-defined nutritional requirements of the horse, but takes those requirements out of the laboratory and thus recognizes that nutrition influences not just the digestive system but all aspects of equine welfare, including behavior; and as well that behavior can influence the eating habits of the horse. It is about using real food to nourish your horse instead of just maintaining his bodily functions and giving him synthetic energy to perform, much as one would lubricate a machine to keep it working. It is about not wasting money plying your horse with every new supplement on the market. Proper nourishment affects more than just the physiological functions of the body; what we all eat, animals included, also affects our other "bodies", being the etheric and astral with respect to non-human animals…but that is a subject reserved for another time. Even though it is long, I consider this a basic instruction in equine nutrition. The basics certainly require some amount of in-depth knowledge of physiology and biochemistry; nutrition can be as much about what not to do as it can what to do. This book does not, however, cover in any detail nutritional treatment of various pathologies that can occur. You will discover, though, that many of these pathologies occur simply because the diet is inappropriate for the species.

This is a statement we have probably all heard in one form or another: "The quality and the convenience of a particular horse feed needs to be weighed against its cost." Where is the aspect of what is best for the horse in this statement? As I undertook an exhaustive amount of research for this book, I found an amazing amount of misdirected information concerning equine nutrition, ranging from vaguely to blatantly erroneous. And not just from lay people, but from professionals as well. And not just from a conventional viewpoint, but from an "alternative" one as well. It is no wonder many people look upon feeding a horse as being a complicated matter! The nutritional requirements for all horses – mares, stallions/geldings, and foals - have not changed in the last 15,000 or so years, since the evolution of the extant Equus caballus species. What has changed is the influence of human involvement and the energy demands that we place upon the horse. Yet the physiological requirements remain the same, and it is when we go against the natural laws under which these requirements were established that we find ourselves facing "problems" that we then try to find ways to "fix" them. My basic philosophy is, when faced with a physical or behavioural problem in a horse, is to first ask "why", and it is from this basic aspect that this book is written. Although much of the equine industry has traditionally demanded that we do so, it is impossible to truly separate other aspects of welfare from nutritional requirements. However, for brevity's sake, I will defer much of the in-depth discussion on specific non-nutritional welfare and behaviour for another book; I wish the reader to understand, however, that aspect is always present even if not in the forefront.

Going up against tradition is never easy. My writings will challenge some long held beliefs and practices, and they may indeed offend some people. It is not my intent to offend, but neither will I dance around the issues. It is, however, my intent to challenge you to think in a light different than the standard cookie cutter one that envelopes today's equine management. What is my purpose in doing so? It's simple…I love horses and I deeply care about their welfare - every aspect of it. The horse/human relationship is evolving and it is my intent and desire to be a significant part of the process. I do not expect everyone to agree with my approach to equine-related issues in this book (and others that I may author), but if this book influences just one person to feed their horse in a manner that is completely appropriate for the species, then I have accomplished my purpose. It is my hope that with the information contained herein at least some horses will be spared the effects of having to wait until something goes amiss with their health before the nutritional aspect is made appropriate. Any more than that is icing on the cake.

We have a chasm between conventional and alternative methodologies. Why? Basically because modern science has evolved into a one-eyed, color blind enigma that can only concentrate on the parts and on making symptoms go away ("if you don't see it, it doesn't exist"). So-called alternatives came along in an attempt to restore some sanity in what was perceived as an insane drive to "dismember" the body in-vivo; in other words, what was perceived as reductionist science. Integrative methodology was born of the effort to "make the best of both worlds" - the only problem is that no one seems to realize that both reside in the same world anyway. The alternative faction offers no real alternative; it is basically the flip side of the same coin as what materialistic, reductionist science is. It is steeped in a nature that it remembers from many centuries past, but it does not really know nature. But what if reductionist science really is valid? Does that invalidate alternative methodologies? To answer both questions: it is valid - if perceived in the correct context; and no, reductionism does not invalidate alternative methods.

There is another science different than either of the above; a perfectly legitimate science that was brought forth many years ago by Johann Wolfgang Von Goethe. It is one that is being rediscovered and recognized today by more than a few enlightened individuals including a number of modern physicists. (Bortoft 1996) It is one that recognizes that separating things into parts does not fracture the whole. The whole is a hologram which is reflected in each part. It is not an entity that is "greater than the sum of its parts" as the alternative faction is fond of saying; that has the tendency to put the whole into a false transcendental position that came before its parts. On the flip side, our typical modern conventional way of thinking is that the whole is an assemblage of interrelated parts, which by definition would make the whole secondary to the parts, the whole being born of the parts. This does not mean that we don't put the parts together, but neither does it mean that the whole only exists because of the parts. Let's take writing for an example. The "whole" of this book as a concept existed before I ever typed the first word. Yet, once it is done, we cannot simply add up all of the words written and get to the whole of the meaning. By the same token, the whole cannot exist realistically without the typed words. It is the specific combination of the parts (the words) that I have put together that (hopefully) conveys to the reader the whole so that the he/she then walks away with an intimate knowing of the whole as opposed to a memorization of parts. This way of knowing is a feeling and participative way of knowing as opposed to an intellectual way of knowing. Both are very valid, and they cannot be separated without losing some of the true underlying meaning of what is being investigated. This is the Goethean holistic way of science. It is every bit as valid applied to any aspect of science, including that of equine nutrition.

It is not my desire to give the student alternatives by only "tinkering with the existing structures" of the current nutritional paradigm as it relates to domestic horses (the phrase in quotes is borrowed from William Brinton in his article "Environment as Data versus "Being": Is Goetheanism possible in the West?"). It is my intent to instill in the student the desire for the ability to create a new paradigm. There is nothing wrong with the biological sciences and chemistry so long as they are approached within the hologram of nature in which they truly exist. By the same token, there is nothing wrong with trying to find "alternatives" to suppressive medicines, and in fact is preferable. An understanding of the former will only naturally lead to a better understanding of the latter if approached from within the context of holistic science.

I have used the male gender term for the biggest part in this book, except where I am specifically referring to mares. The gender terminology is only for simplicity's sake; all things being equal, species appropriate feeding for horses applies to both male and female genders, except as noted in the text.

With regard to references I make about the evolution of horses, this is an area that remains under debate and is changing relatively frequently as more archaeological evidence is uncovered. I have attempted to utilize the latest information as of the current edition of this book.

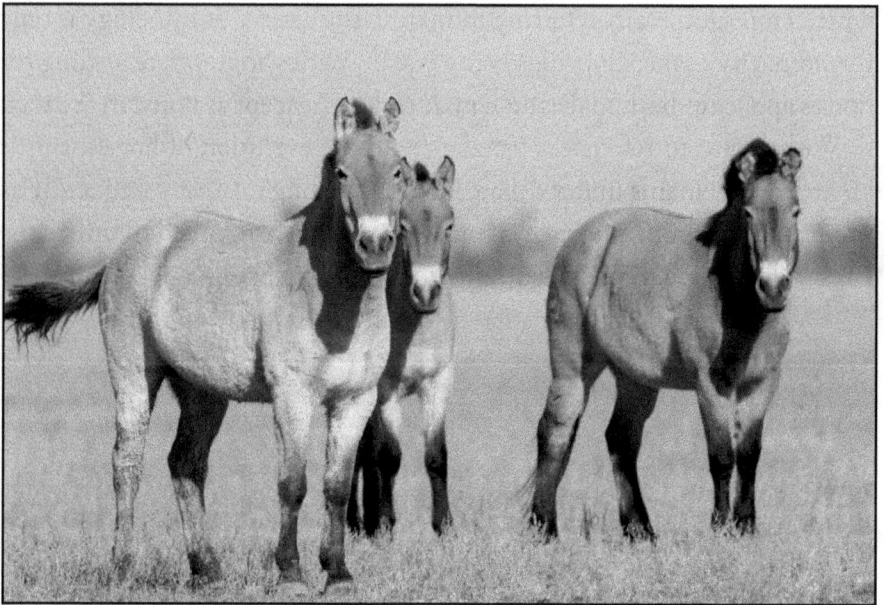

Figure 1: Prezwalski's Horses, Ukrainian steppes in autumn
Source: Shutterstock.com image # 117509296 © Dmytro Pylypenko

Prezwalski's Horse is considered the only true remaining "wild" horse in the world. At one time considered extinct, as of 2011 they are listed as endangered; they live in zoos and reserves throughout the world with the largest breeding program being in the Ukraine.

(Source: http://en.wikipedia.org/wiki/Przewalski's_horse)

2

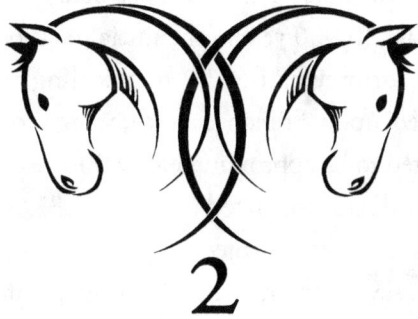

Domestication and the Evolution of Feeding

I N ORDER TO shift the paradigm (to make use of a well-worn cliché) of inappropriate equine feeding, we need to understand why that paradigm exists in the first place. We seem to have gone down the path of accepting as "normal" certain abnormal conditions in our horses. It is "normal" for a racehorse to break down by the time they are 6 or 7, if not earlier (interestingly enough, just about the time they actually physically mature!); bouts of laminitis are almost expected in most horses; colic is way too common as are hoof problems - just to name a few. Changes need to be made if our horses are not to fall prey to external forces beyond their control; which basically means species inappropriate feeding practices and all the problems associated with such practices.

Therefore, it is this author's position that any study of equine nutritional requirements must begin first with a basic understanding of the horse's evolution (to the extent it is currently known) and what effects domestication has had upon feeding practices. It is the impact of physiological evolution that will give us clues as to the nutritive requirements of today's domestic horse. But it is the history of domestication that will give us clues as to why horses are typically fed in the manner that they are today.

Domestication, especially in more recent years, has had a major impact upon the nutrition of the horse. Man has likely had some sort of relationship with Horse for at least 30,000 years. The initial relationship is theorized to have been of a predator/prey nature; i.e. man killing horse for food. This is an assumption based upon French cave drawings found at Lascaux and Pech-Merle, estimated to be approximately 17,000 years BP (before present) and at Chauvet-Pont-d'Arc, estimated to be about 31,000 BP. The paintings frequently show the horse as an object of prey, but they also reveal a sense of majesty that man saw in the horse with the great effort made to recreate the beauty of the horse. (International Museum of the Horse, n.d.)

Then somewhere around 4000-6000 years ago, Equus caballus was brought into domestication, or so it is thought. The exact time frame and the method of domestication are subjects that are still debated, which is interesting given the extreme significance and influence that the horse has had upon human culture. Domestication has traditionally been thought to have occurred over a widespread area in central and Eastern Europe as well as Asia; recent (2009) findings however indicate that the area known as Kazakhstan (once part of the Russian empire and located in central Asia) may have been the first site of domestication of the horse with evidence of uses of riding, food, milk, as well as selective breeding; this is approximately 2000 years prior to known domestication in Europe. (Clarkson 2010) It was once thought that horses died out in North America some 500 years prior to the arrival of humans; however the discovery of horse protein residue on Clovis tools has disputed that theory. Through DNA testing, evidence discovered in 2009 suggests that

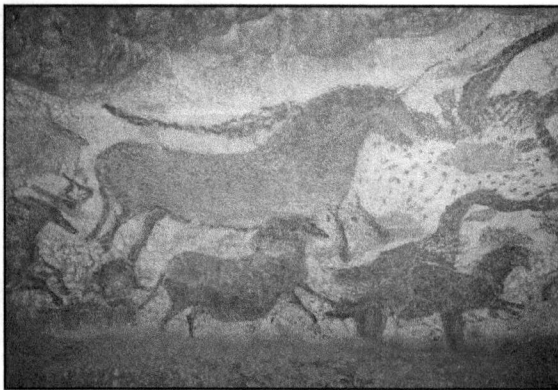

Figure 2: Reproductions of some Lascaux Artworks II
Source: Wikimedia Commons, Jack Versloot 2008

horses survived in North America until only about 7600 years ago, some 5000 years longer than previously thought. (Clarkson 2010) This would create a co-existence timeline between human beings and horses on this continent of over 5000 years. Horses returned to North America in the late 1400's via the Spanish conquistadors, only a few thousand years after their extinction here for reasons that are still being debated. (Clarkson 2010)

Domestication and taming are not the same things. Dr. Bill Jordan, an eminent wildlife advocate and conservationist, defines the two as thus:

> **Domestication** is a process whereby man has structurally, physiologically and behaviourally modified certain species of animals by maintaining them in or near human habitation and by breeding from those certain animals who seem best suited for various human objectives.

> **Taming** is a process whereby a wild animal is subdued into adapting and submitting to human control. Taming of wild animals can be accomplished by various methods but wildness is still there and can be triggered off by undue stress. (Jordan 2003)

A domesticated animal will give birth to tame offspring; a tame animal will not necessarily give birth to tame offspring. The accepted definition of domestication is a bit tricky in this author's opinion. Does domestication truly change the physiology of the species? Some say that the domestication of dog has turned him into an omnivore. If this is true, then why did not his dentition change to reflect that? The pressure of domestication and intentional breeding may indeed change some physical traits (the structure), but to say that the underlying physiological function of the species has changed is, in my opinion, simply not true. Only through modifying the genotype can that be accomplished (which is certainly being attempted with some life forms). Behavior can become modified in a domestication process for many various reasons, but is it truly permanently altered? There is likely not a horse existing that, if returned to feral conditions, would not revert to undomesticated behavior, including dietary patterns. Either that or we have not ever truly domesticated the horse!

Therefore, the singular act of domestication alone does not create a physiological change in overall nutritional requirements; in other words, domesticating a horse does not change his requirement to forage for food over the greater part of a 24-hour period into one in which he is physiologically adapted to eating two or three meals per day. A change of that magnitude would require a substantial change in anatomy and physiology that can only naturally be brought about by extensive periods of evolutionary mutation. Changes in nutrient ratios and quantities can, however, affect some physical traits such as size. To wit, the feral island ponies of Assateague Island, Maryland: they rarely reach thirteen hands in their wild environment even though they are descended from full sized horses, but if a foal is removed and fed a high protein diet, he will grow to what we think of as "normal" for an average domesticated horse. (Olsen 2003) (p 66)

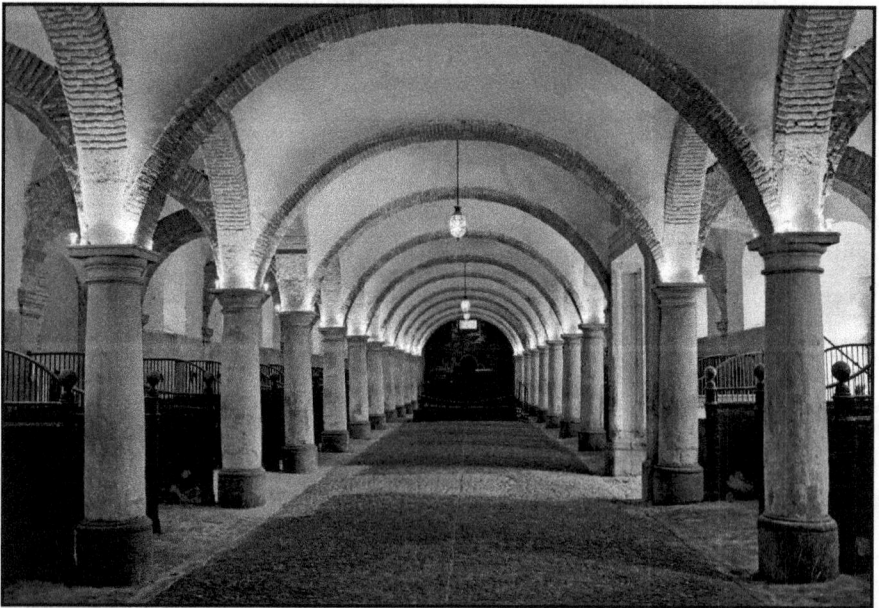

Figure 3: Arched interior of the 16th century Royal Stables in Cordoba, Andalusia, Spain.
Source: Shutterstock.com image # 108160277 © Artur Bogacki

Truly wild horses are almost non-existent (see photo plate preceding this chapter); the so-called "wild" Mustangs of western North America are feral, being descendants of domesticated horses that were bred for ease of handling. According to Anthony, truly wild horses are alert and suspicious, and may be aggressive. (Olsen 2003 #33 (p 67) [Anthony's definition of aggressive may be subjective in this author's opinion, and we would have to know exactly how he defines this; being alert and suspicious is not an uncommon trait for even domestic horses.] One has to wonder why horses were domesticated in the first place: Anthony suggests it was because of their greater adaptability in snowy conditions than other already domesticated farm animals such as cattle, sheep, and pigs –meaning they were kept for human food purposes. (Olsen 2003 #33 (pp 67-68) The act of domestication by human beings can, however, heavily influence the feeding practices of a given animal species, especially combined with the so-called "advances" in the science of fractionated nutrition. Domestication eventually brought about the practice of stabling horses which effectively prevented them from foraging their own food, at least the part of the day they were kept up. One of the earliest known stables was found in Egypt and was estimated to have existed over 3000 years ago. (Anna 2008) Many of these stables, especially those of the wealthy, were architectural marvels in themselves, much more grand that most people's homes are even today.

The advent of stabling as well as the evolving "use" of horses under human direction had a tremendous impact upon feeding practices, although these practices did and still do vary greatly from one part of the world to another.

The horse has played an integral role in human culture from the moment human had first contact with horse, whenever that may have been. Equestrian sporting activities have existed since at least ancient Roman and Grecian empires, with horse racing becoming an established professional sport by the early 1700's. While the initial stages of the industrial revolution actually brought about an increase in work for horses, including even more varied jobs (American Museum of Natural History), the machine age eventually caused a decisive shift in the human-equine relationship. No longer were horses needed for mobility purposes and their job as farm workers declined to the point that today we typically only see novel uses of horses working on the farm. The decreasing importance of the horse in overall human culture within the United States from about 1918 up until the 1960's led to a decline in equine research – including nutrition – at universities and agricultural stations. (Hintz and Cymbaluk 1994) The 1960's saw a resurgence of the use of horses in human culture, but this time with much more emphasis on pleasure and sporting activities. As universities and colleges here re-instituted equine research programs, we began to see a shift in feeding practices with the advent of more "scientific" feeds formulated for specific levels of activity, from pleasure to racing and eventing. Prior to the 1960's, most "advances" in equine nutrition occurred in Europe, primarily the United Kingdom, and working horses were mostly fed a diet of cereal grains such as oats and boiled barley, the exact feed constituents being geographically dependent. Although some appeared on the market before, it was primarily after the 1960's and the expansion of the development of concentrates for various activity levels that horses began being fed highly processed feeds. Appendix 1 contains a brief timeline of some of the more significant introductions in equine feeds. It is interesting to see that by the later 1980's feed companies began in earnest concentrating on trying to "fix" hoof problems with nutrition, with laminitis coming into full view by the early 1990's.

As science moved more and more into the materialistic and reductionist realm, we saw the introduction of fortified feeds, also known as compound feeds. The conventional view of nutritional science has this tendency to believe that anything found in nature can be made in a laboratory and be just as effective, or even better. While these individual synthetic substances (vitamins and minerals) may have the same chemical structure as their natural counterparts, they lack the synergistic effects of the constituents found in nature, and more importantly, the natural enzyme catalysts. Synthetic vitamins and minerals lack the bioavailability of those found in nature. According to Wikipedia (Wikipedia 2007): "Compound feeds are feedstuffs that are blended from various raw materials and additives. These blends are formulated according to the specific requirements of the target animal. They are manufactured by feed compounders as meal type, pellets or crumbles." Primary types of compound feed are the "concentrates", being low in fiber but high in carbohydrates, proteins, and fats, and formulated to deliver varying degrees of calories.

The first question to ask is why are we taking raw products that may be a horse's natural food with naturally bioavailable nutrients, cooking them thus devoiding them of their intrinsic nutrients, then adding the synthetic version back in (not to mention the preservatives now needed) and then feeding this concoction to the horse? Would it not be easier to allow the horse to obtain his own food as nature intended? Where is the evidence that horses who are allowed to forage their own food are calorie deficient? The answers appear to be complicated, but I think if we take this step by step we can begin to realize that feeding horses is not – and should not be – as complicated as the equine feed industry would have us believe. Obviously domesticated use of the horse has been a huge influence in the attempt to bring a higher caloric intake to horses, especially once horses began to be used in physically demanding sports. Nevertheless, these are living, breathing, sentient beings, not machines that we feed "fuel" to so they can operate faster. Uncomplicating the feeding process for horses is multi-faceted; we are going to have to look beyond just their physiological needs if we are to come to an understanding that allows the horse to live in a domestic situation that is both ethologically sound and healthy for him. Getting to this understanding will require a complete change in thinking about domestic horses for many people…and a change in many of the entrenched practices.

Some of the primary reasons for the way domestic horses have been and continue to be fed lie with owner convenience and deeply entrenched feeding practices that that seem to have been birthed out of anthropocentrism. In fairly recent history but prior to the industrial revolution, at the end of a long day of work, horses were brought back to the stable and given their meal of (likely) oats and/or bran mash, and "put to bed". But they were also typically fed during the work day when the human would take breaks, resulting in a few to several feedings during a 24 hour period instead of the standard one or two we find today. Additionally, much of the horses' grain-type feed at that time was either grown by the farmer or at least was obtained locally, and it was clean (meaning not having chemicals applied), whole grain high in fiber. And that is not to say even that was an entirely species appropriate diet. This feeding practice has survived for centuries with the modification that horses today are generally only fed once or twice per day. And instead of a single type of grain, they are now given concoctions of different fortified grains (many of which are now genetically modified) with perhaps some herbs thrown in to make us feel like we are doing something really good for our horse, not to mention a multitude of supplements for various perceived reasons. Some of the more fortunate horses are also allowed access to pasture in varying degrees, which should theoretically cut down on the amount of compound feed they are given although many times in practice it makes no difference. Interestingly, a small study was done in 2011 that indicated horses that were allowed only restricted access to pasture during a 24 hour period actually were able to consume more grass on a percentage basis during that time (3 hours) than the control group that was allowed pasture access the entire 24 hours period. (Andrews 2011) So what we wind up with are horses that have been overfed and/or improperly fed for generations. And, although definitive information is lacking, it is curious to think that the basis for the initial domestication of the horse might have been the original influencing factor upon our current feeding practices. In other words, if humans did indeed originally domesticate horses for food purposes, would they not have wanted to "fatten" them up prior to slaughter? If so, has this practice become so entrenched in our historical association with horses that we lost conscious thought about it thousands of years ago? And in more recent times, what metabolic effect has the extensive use of processed feeds had on horses? We are certainly seeing detrimental effects on humans that eat too much processed foods. Could these species inappropriate feeding practices be contributing to a generational effect of metabolic abnormalities which we are now seeing an "epidemic" of?

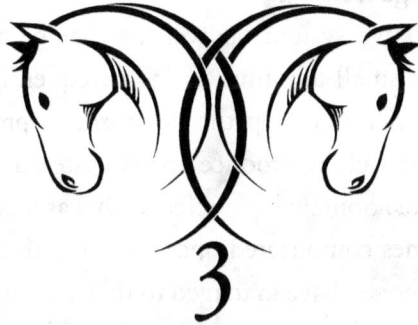

3
THE PHYSIOLOGY OF EQUINE DIGESTION

H AVING EVOLVED OVER a long period of time to become the physiological entities they are today, horses are classified as ungulate mammals, which are large bodied herbivores. An herbivore is an animal that primarily feeds on herbaceous (non-woody) vegetation. There are two types of herbivores. One type includes the ruminants (such as cattle, sheep and goats) that have a compartmentalized stomach, the first compartment of which is called the rumen. The second type, known as non-ruminant herbivores, includes horses, rabbits and rats, as well as hippopotamus and rhinoceros; these animals have a significantly-sized large intestine which includes what is known as a "functional caecum". The rumen in ruminants acts as a fermentation vat in which billions of microbes do the job of breaking down the tough fibrous plant material. The caecum in the latter type of herbivore is where the microbes do their job of fermenting and breaking down the structural fiber into nutrients that can be assimilated. The difference being that in ruminants, this fermentation process takes place toward the beginning of the digestive system, and in horses it takes place toward the end. Thus, horses are known as "hindgut fermenters" and need larger overall quantities of forages than ruminants do to produce the same amount of calories – but as we shall see, it is imperative this caloric intake occurs on an almost continual basis in horses and not from infrequent, large feedings.

The horse's digestive system (as well as that of other herbivores) is designed to process small amounts of food frequently, converting them into available nutrients that keep the organism in proper working order (i.e., homeostasis) as well as produce appropriate amounts of energy for various life functions. Some people refer to this as a complicated process. It really only becomes complicated once we bring domestication into the picture. Obviously horses have managed to thrive quite well as a species on their own for millions of years with no input from humans. Before we look at how domestication complicates this process in the summation chapter, let's first examine the digestive system so we have a good understanding of why the horse needs to eat these small amounts of herbaceous plants frequently – what we commonly call a "trickle feeder"; after that we will go through the basic nutrient requirements.

3.1 Mouth

The mouth, also known as the oral cavity, is the obvious place to begin. If you've ever closely watched a horse grazing in a natural environment, you would have seen him use both his keen senses of smell and touch to determine what plants to eat. Horses have prehensile, upper lips that are used to select specific forages for consumption; these same lips act as a funnel when drinking water. Their upper and lower incisors (the front teeth) are used to snip forages off at various proximities to the ground, generally no greater than about two inches; they then use their tongues to move the plant material to the cheek teeth (premolars and molars) where the matter is ground up using a circular type of chewing motion, known as mastication. This chewing motion helps to begin the process of breaking down the fibrous plant material into nutrients that can be later assimilated. A horse has 3 pairs of salivary glands which produce up to 12 liters (3 gallons) of mucus containing saliva through the parotid gland daily. (Kentucky Equine Research Staff 2011b) This is based on a species appropriate diet of natural forages;

grain meals produce significantly less saliva, with sweet feed producing almost no saliva. This aspect is likely where the practice of giving a small amount of apple cider with feed got its start as the cider vinegar helps to both stimulate saliva production when being fed concentrates as well as increase the buffering. (Kohnke 2008) The horse generally does not begin to salivate on anticipation of food, but primarily when the food is in the mouth. This saliva wets and lubricates the forage, and also contains bicarbonate, which serves to buffer the high acidity of the stomach. Salivary amylase, an enzyme that hydrolyzes starches into sugars,

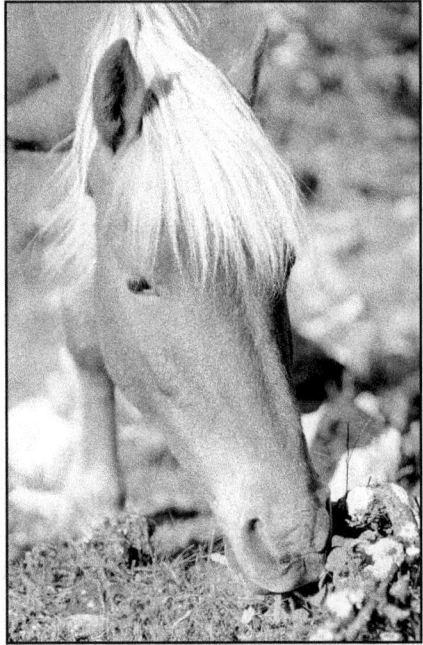

Figure 4: Horse grazing
Source: Shutterstock.com image # 77212840;
© neneo

is found in very small to non-existent amounts in the equine mouth. (Burk 2009), (Macleod 2007), (Sellnow 2006) [This fact has been used to indicate that horses are not adapted to eating starch; however what is not being taken into consideration is the amount of amylase present in raw food. We find this according to Dr. Cichoke in his book, The Complete Book of Enzyme Therapy: "Although amylase is found in nongreen tissues and organs, it is almost always found in the green parts of plants." (Cichoke 1998) Therefore, if the horse is getting a natural forage based diet, he should get sufficient amylase to support pre-digestion of starches found in such forage.] As indicated above, on a dry matter basis, a horse eating at pasture and/or hay will produce twice the amount of saliva as when he eats grain or concentrates. Therefore, diets high in grain/concentrates and low in forages will result in lower gastric pH values, potentiating the risk for ulcerative conditions.

Obviously proper chewing of the food is vital and thus maintaining proper dental care is important in this process. But horses that are allowed access to pasture 24/7 along with hay as needed and whose diets do not consist primarily of concentrates will not tend as frequently to get the sharp edges that can hinder eating for two reasons: one is the varying silica content in natural forages that tend to keep the teeth worn down, and the other is the full-jaw sweeping motion that the horse takes when grazing. (Sellnow 2006) It is interesting to note that horses have hypsodont dentition, meaning their teeth (incisors, premolars, and molars) "erupt" over their lifetime. In other words, there is only a certain amount of tooth that any horse is ever going to have. As the horse wears the grinding surface down from eating, the tooth erupts from the gum until there is no crown remaining, generally at a rate of about 1/8" per year; of course this will vary with the diet. This is what can make feeding old horses a bit of a challenge; a horse that is 15-20 years or older may begin to lose some teeth naturally. (See the sub-chapter on Feeding the Senior Horse for more information.)

Another aspect of feeding that should be noted here is that of proximity to the ground. Horses are physiologically designed to eat at ground level, not out of a bucket or hay net hanging several feet off the ground. Feeding at a level higher than a few inches off the ground can cause choke.

This is an interesting table of how many "chews" a horse will take before he swallows his food:

Hay (dry, long stem)*	3500-4500 chews/kg	Long chaff is chewed into finer particles than is short chop chaff
Oats	800-1000 chews/kg	
Sweet Feed (concentrate)	350-500 chews/kg	Note there is greatly reduced chewing resulting in rapid consumption and less saliva buffering
Feed Pellets + mash	400-480 chews/kg	Ditto

* I was not able to find data on haylage   (kg = 2.2 lbs)

Figure 5: Table of number of chews in various feeds
Information sources: http://www.kohnkesown.com/digestion.pdf &
http://www.aaep.org/health_articles_view.php?id=200

When we compare the hindgut fermentation of the horse to that of a foregut fermenter, such as the cow, we find that the horse necessarily has a more rapid transit time through the foregut and therefore is less efficient at cellulose digestion, which is compensated for in the greater quantity of food required. Not having the regurgitation capability that foregut fermenters do, it is also necessary that the cell content of the plant material must be accessible prior to arrival in the fermentation vat. (Fletcher *et al.* 2010) This latter aspect is hypothesized as the reason that horses will chew forages to the relatively great extent that they do.

3.2 Esophagus

The esophagus is the next stop along the digestive tract. It is a simple muscular tube that typically measures four to five feet in length. As the esophagus empties into the stomach we find something called the cardiac sphincter, which is a muscular ring that is extremely well developed in horses and has the ability to shut tight. This combined with the oblique angle at which the esophagus enters the stomach explains why a horse cannot in most cases vomit, although any food remaining in the esophagus can be regurgitated to some degree. The esophagus is also the area where horses can experience choke. Horses that are fed an unnatural diet of processed feeds can sometimes "bolt" their feed (eat too fast) which can lead to choke. This can also apply to stalled horses that are let out to pasture infrequently. Crunchy type foods such as carrots, apples, etc can cause choking issues if they are not chewed properly. So it is always wise when feeding these types of treats to make sure they are a proper size for the particular horse to be able to masticate fully. The senior horse that has very few teeth left should not be fed crunchy type treats…use softer cookies, etc made for horses

3.3 STOMACH

The equine stomach is a J-shaped organ that is capable of holding and mixing up to only about three to four gallons of digesta at a time. The stomach's size relative to the body is indicative of a species that is known as a trickle feeder. The stomach has some elasticity, but if it becomes too distended (gastric dilatation), it can quickly lead to gastric rupture if not treated right away. Causes of gastric dilatation include ingesting a single large meal especially one containing large amounts of fermentable foodstuff such as grain, lush grasses that the horse is not adapted to, and/or beet pulp; it is presumed that the large increase in volatile fatty acids inhibit gastric emptying. (Kahn 2010) Therefore, the equine stomach works best when it has frequent passage of food into it and the rate of passage through it is, under normal circumstances, dictated by the volume. Fiber-based digesta typically moves through the stomach quite rapidly (about 20 minutes), and many times it is leaving the stomach via the pyloric valve as food is entering the stomach from the esophagus (assuming the horse has free choice access to a natural food supply). Since the stomach normally empties when it is about two-thirds full (a protective mechanism against the inability to vomit), the larger the meal or the smaller the particles, the quicker it will also move through the foregut, effectively cutting down nutrient absorption if the rate of passage is excessive. Heavy, dense grains and high protein meals will have a tendency to accumulate in the lower glandular portion of the stomach. Gastric acid is produced at variable continual rates and is not dependent upon eating with the caveat that the acid production ceases after prolonged periods of fasting (48 hours or more). (Lardy and Poland 2001), (Macleod 2007), (Kohnke 2008), (Wikipedia 2012) Furthermore, it appears that this acid variability in at least the adult horse is caused more by duodenal reflux than saliva especially when the stomach is relatively empty. Since the reflux contents contain high sodium and bicarbonate concentrations, the reflux action provides an extra measure of protection against the acid environment of the stomach. This process is apparently not fully understood, but this duodenal reflux does seem to be a natural function of the horse as endoscopic observation shows that the pyloric sphincter in the horse is open most of the time. (Mende n.d.) It is also of interest to note that the administration of histamine-2 blocking agents has been shown to significantly inhibit gastric acid secretion since the natural secretion itself is triggered by the interaction of endogenous histamine in the first place. (Merritt 2003a)

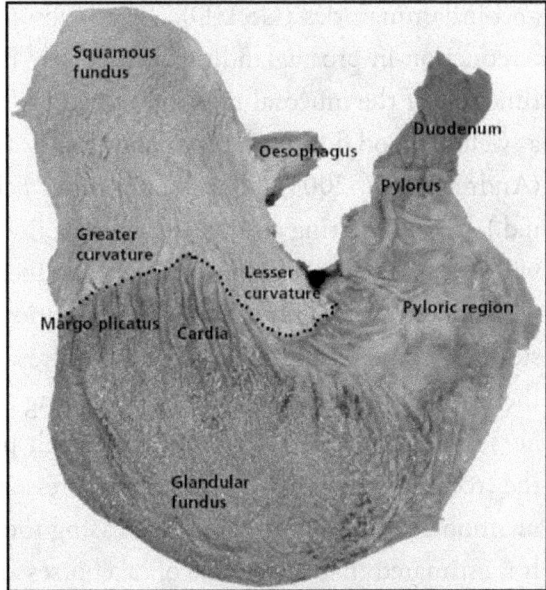

Figure 6: Equine stomach/upper & lower sections
Source: www.atlantaequine.com

The stomach consists of two distinct sections divided by what is known as the margo plicatus. Ingesta enters the stomach from the esophagus in the proximal non-glandular, or saccus caecus, portion of the stomach which is lined with squamous epithelium, and thus only minimally protected from gastric acids. The majority of equine stomach ulcers will occur in this region. (Andrews *et al.* 2005) The distal portion of the stomach, consisting of the fundic and pyloric regions, is a glandular one lined with mucus membranes that secrete not only bicarbonate-rich mucus but the hydrochloric acids and pepsinogen necessary for the initial stages of digestion. The pH of this region can dip very low, to 2.6. (Macleod 2007) [Note that it is possible for the pH to drop even lower as was demonstrated in 1993 by Baker and Gerring (Merritt 2003b).] Gastric ulcers in the distal portion are typically of low occurrence [at least according to Merritt when he wrote his article; the infrequency of occurrence may be debatable some nine years later] and can happen when a breakdown of the protective barrier happens due to stress-induced release of endogenous cortisol and/or the administration of non-steroidal anti-inflammatories (NSAID). These substances (the NSAID) can cause a reduction in prostaglandins (particularly PGE-2), thereby reducing the function of the mucosal membrane and of the production of bicarbonate as well as blood flow to the epithelium; they also increase HCl production. (Andrews *et al.* 2005), (Tuft's Cummings School of Veterinary Medicine n.d.) It is interesting to note that corn oil at a rate of about 45 mL/day will decrease gastric acid production and increase the production of prostaglandins. Diets with a high calcium ratio may also serve to buffer the stomach contents and increase pH. (Andrews *et al.* 2005) I believe this is the very reason that the practice of feeding corn oil is so prevalent in the horse industry, especially within the high performance sector, allowing the frequent usage of NSAID for the stressed horse's musculature (not to mention actual injuries) while decreasing the occurrence of gastric ulcers. It is estimated that up to 90% of racehorses and up to 60% of show horses will feel the effects of equine gastric ulcers. (Frederickson and Noordergraaf 2006) Recent research has shown that the horse can digestively handle dietary fat to a higher degree than previously thought, with no seeming adverse effects. The point is, though, that we should not be using dietary fat as a crutch to continue practices that are ultimately detrimental to the horse's welfare.

It is well known that ruminants (cows, goats, etc) have very active fermentation processes in the foregut, however many people do not associate foregut fermentation with monogastric herbivores. It has long been assumed that the acidic environment of the equine stomach was not conducive to microbial fermentation. Even though structural carbohydrate fermentation processes actively take place in the hindgut, research within the past several years has shown there is considerable bacterial fermentation of sugar and starch in the equine stomach before the ingesta passes through to the small intestine, the extent being dependent upon the composition of the diet. In a presentation made by A. M. Merritt to the Association of Equine Practitioners in 2003 and based upon research first done in the 1940's and especially that reported in a 1963 paper by Alexander and Davies, he states that intra-gastric fermentation of carbohydrates is significant under certain dietary conditions. Lactobacillus acidophilus and Streptococcus bovis have the capability of surviving well in a relatively acidic environment. The by-product of the fermentation activity of these microbes is lactic acid and can reach fairly high proportions if there is a significant quantity of soluble carbohydrates. (Merritt 2003a) The microbes that ferment carbohydrates into volatile fatty acids (VFAs) are indeed more pH sensitive, which is why they are found in high numbers in the hindgut, however there is evidence they are also present in the equine stomach. Merritt hypothesizes that "they colonize within the coarser fibrous ingesta, which collects towards the top of the stratified mat of gastric contents, where the pH of the contents is more to their liking because the mat has not been fully penetrated by gastric acid". He further states that the VFAs produced in the horse's stomach are not absorbed into the bloodstream via the gastric wall. While it has been demonstrated that the cessation of strenuous training (i.e. reduction of stress) can stop and actually resolve gastric lesions found in the fundic region, it appears to be more likely that the intra-gastric fermentation of soluble carbohydrates and the resulting VFA production is the etiological link to squamous gastritis, as has been demonstrated by the use of antacids resulting in lesion regression even when the horse was kept in strenuous training. (Merritt 2003b) Of course performance horses have traditionally been fed a diet high in soluble carbohydrates in the form of concentrates to boost their energy levels; therefore you have the combination of both stress and high levels of soluble carbs.

There is also non-fermentative digestion in the equine stomach; two digestive gastric enzymes produced by zymogen cells have been noted in particular in the horse – pepsin and lipase, and this is in concordance with most mammalian species. Pepsin functions as a proteolytic (breaks down proteins) in an acid medium (conversion to pepsin occurs at pH < 4.0), and while there is more than one form of pepsinogen in the equine stomach, there does not seem to be any data showing the extent to which pepsin functions in protein digestion in the horse's stomach (i.e. how much dietary protein is actually absorbed from gastric digestion). The same situation exists for lipase, which has the function of digesting fats; and horses appear to produce a large amount of gastric lipase, but again, the exact digestive function – or the extent of it - upon the ingesta is not known. (Merritt 2003a)

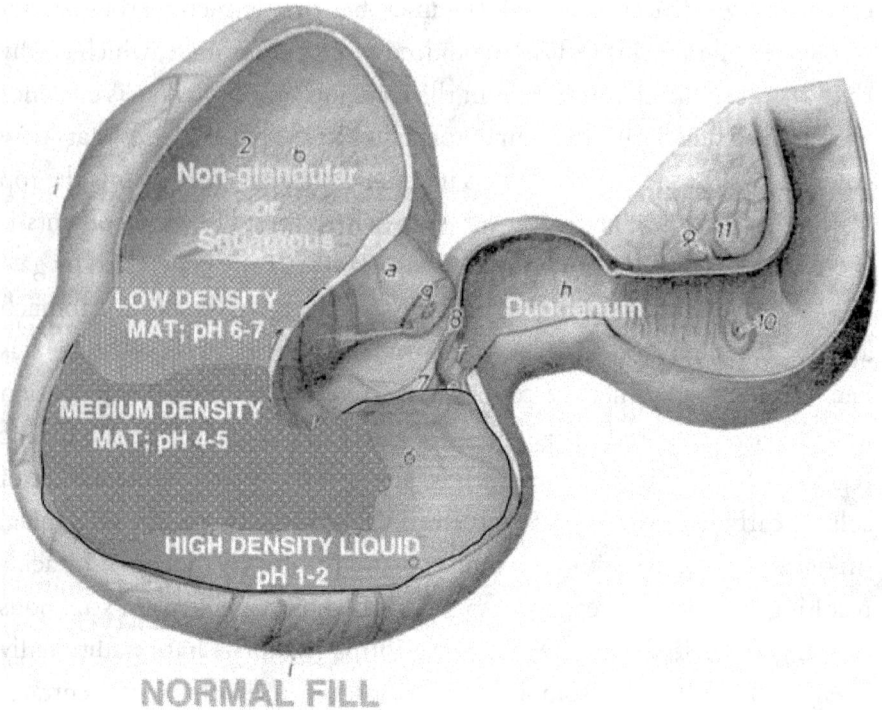

Figure 7: Equine Stomach/fill rates
Source: The Equine Stomach: A Personal Perspective (1963-2003), Merritt, A.M., IVIS.org; As presented to the 49th Annual Convention of AAEP, 2003

Even though the above figure is labeled "normal", according to Dr. Merritt (via email 12/04/2012), it "might represent what is found in a horse confined to a stall with hay available free-choice and grain given twice daily". Therefore we cannot truly label this as normal as defined as a horse that is not stalled and allowed his natural diet of free-access forage with no forced meals. Dr. Merritt goes on to state that "the contents in a horse that is eating primarily roughage on the free-choice basis will be more consistently fibrous throughout, and the overall fill will be greater". In all cases, though, the pH gradient remains, the degree of which can be altered by exercise and feeding patterns.

It is my opinion that the "take-home" message from the horse having foregut (specifically gastric) fermentation capability is that the purpose is to "pre-digest" non-structural carbohydrates, at a level that is typically found in a raw foraging diet. Accordingly, it is my further thought that this capability is inherent for reasons related to the horse's natural dietary needs: intact forages will tend to fluctuate in sugar and starch levels both diurnally and seasonally. This fermentation capability, again in my opinion, is an evolutionary design mechanism that facilitates these fluctuations. It is when the levels of soluble carbs – especially those that are derived from processed sources - reach proportions greater than the stomach is designed to digestively handle that we begin seeing an abnormal amount of fermentation with the resulting potential of the Equine Gastric Ulcer Syndrome (EGUS) condition that seems to plague performance horses and those in training especially, and which can certainly include those horses that are stalled and fed infrequently. Masking or suppressing the symptoms of EGUS with drugs is not resolving the problem, and is nothing more than a situation of pandering to industry demands. Therefore, while I do believe that performance horses can perform quite well on a "raw" diet to a certain extent we also have to ask some hard questions as to whether or not our "use" of horses is for their benefit or ours, and how can we come to a *mutually* beneficial existence in which their physiological needs are completely respected.

With regard to the non-fermentative enzyme digestive capability in the stomach, I feel there are some clues yet to be discovered relative to the equine digestive process. The presence of pepsinogen is not terribly surprising as there is a certain amount of protein in all forages of varying degree. It is the "large" amount of gastric lipase that I find very curious as the horse's natural diet does not, supposedly, contain significant amounts of dietary fat.

3.4 Small Intestine

The digesta now moves out of the stomach, passing through the duodenum via the pyloric sphincter. Without a gall bladder, bile is secreted by the duodenal glands and liver, which is done continuously (with the exception that after a 48 hour fast, bile secretion ceases) along with bicarbonates in order to neutralize the pH of the digesta; there is also a protective mucosal covering. This neutralization process is necessary as pancreatic and intestinal enzymes can only work in a neutral or slightly alkaline environment as opposed to the plant enzymes which can function in a very wide pH range. Transit time through the small intestine is variable but typically rapid; some digesta will normally begin to appear in the caecum after approximately 45 minutes of digestion time in the small intestine. (Macleod 2007) The shorter the time spent in the small intestine, the fewer nutrients are absorbed. Note that processed feeds (pelleted and ground feeds) as well as large grain meals will move quicker through the small intestine than will fibrous feeds. Exercise can also decrease transit time. (Geor 2002)

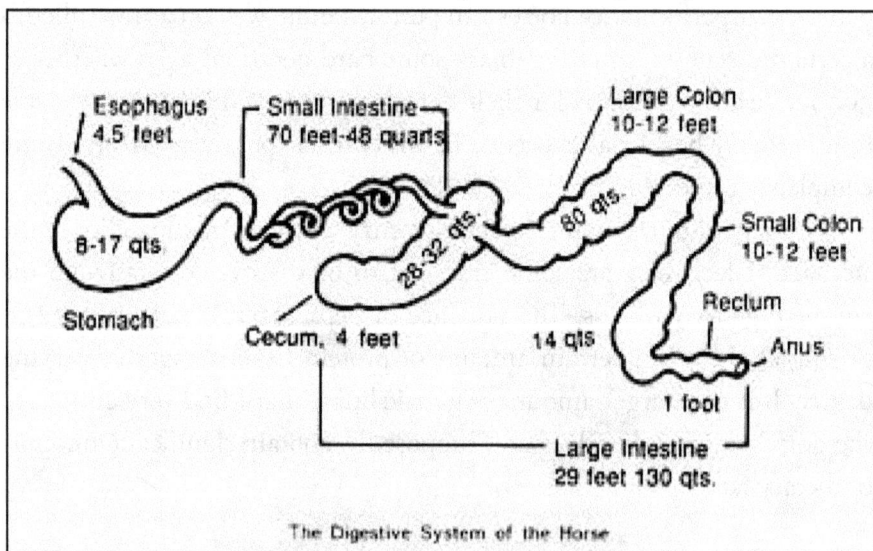

Figure 8: Equine digestive tract/Ohio State
Source: OHIO STATE UNIV, BULLETIN 762-00

The small intestine, consisting of the duodenum, jejunum, and the ileum, represents about twenty-eight percent of the horse's digestive systems and is relatively small given the horse's size; if you were to extend it, it would measure approximately 70 feet in length and about three to four inches in diameter. The small intestine can hold approximately twelve+ gallons. This is where serious digestion takes place via the enzymatic processes that allow nutrient absorption by catalyzing chemical reactions. Proteins, lipids (fats and oils), non-structural carbohydrates (sugars and starches), amino acids, minerals and vitamins are digested well in the small intestine; the villi found in the surface area of the small intestine aid nutrient absorption into the bloodstream. The carbohydrates that are processed here are broken down into glucose molecules that provide necessary energy to the cells via the action of insulin. While the small intestine supplies some digestive enzymes, most of them come from the pancreas (which also produces the insulin hormone). The pancreas secretes enzymatic juices continuously in small amounts with an increase in production in response to the arrival of digesta. Horses apparently have comparatively low concentrations of pancreatic amylase suggesting a limited ability to digest starches (non-structural polysaccharides); according to Macleod, the amylase concentration in horses is about half that of the pig, although there can be wide individual variations (see the discussion on Polysaccharides in Chapter 3.2). She says that all grains, other than oats, should be processed prior to feeding in order to increase starch digestibility. (Macleod 2007) This is corroborated via tests done by Kentucky Equine Research (KER). All starches are made up of chains of glucose however the architecture of those chains is what impacts the digestibility of the various grains. Their tests showed that oats had the most prececal digestibility, followed by sorghum, corn, and barley. (Pagan 1998a) Hoffman also corroborates this stating that if the starch is contained within whole grains that have waxy seed coats (e.g. rice or corn) or within rigid cell walls (e.g. whole soybean), this can inhibit the ability of pancreatic amylase to access and break the starches down; milling and grinding will increase the susceptibility to the hydrolyzation process necessary for the digestion of starches. (Hoffman 2003)[1]

On the other hand, horses do produce significant amounts of sugar-digesting enzymes, (Macleod 2007) indicating that dietary sugar – given a natural diet and proper lifestyle – should not pose any metabolic issues for horses. It does not, however, indicate that sweet feed or other processed sugars are good for the horse. Again, we are talking about a biophysical process, not just a biochemical one. The actual fibrous (cell wall) components of forages are not digested very well in the small intestine and flow to the next section (the caecum and remainder of large intestine).

Ruminants have somewhat of a detoxifying capability in their foregut given the large amount of fermentation that naturally occurs, which may be why you find many cattle owners not terribly worried about feeding moldy hay (to an extent - there is, of course, a limit that even cows can handle). Horses, being primarily hindgut fermenters, do not have this opportunity to detoxify substances prior to entry into the small intestine. Therefore with the small intestine being the primary site of nutrient absorption, it has the potential to also transport toxins into the bloodstream. While most of us might typically think of "toxins" as being poisonous plants or other substances, we would not necessarily think of a normal feed as being toxic. However, keep in mind that whatever is put into that feed is absorbed into the bloodstream, and that includes chemical preservatives found in almost all processed feeds. These substances then become toxins that the emunctories have to deal with, especially the liver. The only saving grace in this aspect may be that, as stated above, processed feeds tend to

---

[1] Another aspect of whole grain indigestibility is that some people assume there is lack of digestion when they see grain hulls in the horse's manure; this is not necessarily true and can mean that processing negates visible fibrous material in the manure – it does not necessarily have a direct correlation to digestion of nutrients (including the breakdown of starches) within the grain and simply means that the hulls alone are not very digestible. (Coleman 2001) Most studies with regard to whether grains for horses should be processed or not seem to be concerned primarily with net energy gain versus cost of processing, with the conclusion that the processing of oats primarily has little benefit; not the same for other grains such as barley, and corn especially requiring grinding and/or heat processing . (Coleman 2001) Oats, being a soft grain, can be masticated in the horse's mouth much easier than hard grains. It does not seem apparent, however, that there was any thought given to plant based enzyme inhibitors in whole grains in the studies I saw, including oats: human research shows that raw grains (as well as nuts and beans for human consumption) contain enzyme inhibitors. (Lee et al. 1998)

move quicker through the small intestine with less absorption. However, this does not mean they are always "safe" with regard to chemicals they contain as there can be adverse effects within the large intestine, let alone a compounding effect.

Our modern use of horses practically demands that feed pass through the digestive tract as quickly as possible so that the horse may be returned to whatever work regimen the owner sees fit, and the feed companies have been more than obliging. The resulting digestive complications then become fodder for pharmaceutical companies.

3.5 Large Intestine

Up to this point we have been investigating what is commonly known as the "foregut" of the horse. After leaving the small intestine, digesta enters the caecum, the first part of the "hindgut" of the horse. From the time of ingestion, food begins to arrive in the hindgut typically within one to three hours. The caecum, located in the right flank area, makes up the first part of the large intestine, and is where the bulk of the fermentation processes take place. The other four parts of the large intestine are the large colon, small colon, rectum, and anus. [Note that some sources do not include the anus when discussing the large intestine, leaving the remaining four parts; furthermore some sources combine the large and small colon into one, calling it "the colon"; and to add even more confusion, yet other references will call the two colons the large intestine, referring to the caecum as part of the hind gut but not part of the large intestine per se.] As you can see from the diagram above (Figure 8), the entire colon (large and small) consists of ascending, transverse, and descending parts. The large colon is the ascending part; the small colon is the descending part. The main parts of the large intestine comprise over 60% of the horse's entire digestive system, and complete digestion here will normally take a couple of days or slightly longer.

Type	Foregut	Capacity (apprx)	Pct of GIT
Enzymatic Digestion (small intestine primarily; some fermentative digestion in stomach)	Stomach	2-4 gallons	8%
	Small Intestine	12-17 gallons	30%
Type	Hindgut	Capacity (apprx)	Pct of GIT
Microbial Digestion	Caecum	7-10 gallons	15%
	Large Colon	20+ gallons	38%
	Small Colon	3.5-4 gallons	9%

Figure 9: Table of Foregut vs Hindgut digestive capabilities
Source: Adapted from *Atlas of Topographical Anatomy of the Domestic Animals*;
Popesko, P; Saunders, W.B.

The caecum is a sac approximately three to four feet long; it can hold roughly between seven and ten gallons of food and liquid depending upon the size of the (adult) horse. It empties into the right ventral colon and right and left distal colon, which are joined by flexures (narrow bends). The caecum and colon have pouch-like structures called sacculations which, along with the flexures, separate the entire the hindgut into compartments that aid in the fermentation process. (Macleod 2007) Digesta flows from the caecum to the large colon, then into the small colon. The small colon is responsible for reclaiming excess moisture, returning it to the body, which results in fecal balls being formed and which are then passed into the rectum for eventual expulsion from the anus. (Sellnow 2006) Peristalsis is the mechanism by which digesta is moved through the entire large intestine. It normally takes at least 24 hours before an ingested meal starts to come out at the other end as droppings. However, this rate is variable, with most waste from a particular meal having been excreted within about 65 hours [some references say up to 72 hours]. The excrements will consist of varying amounts of water, feed residue, digestive secretions, epithelial cells, salts, bacteria, and the end products of the fermentation process. (Macleod 2007) If the horse is allowed to trickle feed as it should, there will likely be both "old" and "new" foodstuff in the caecum at the same time.

Looking back at Figure 8, we can see at least a couple of potential places for colic in the horse's large intestine. One is the caecum itself. Being a "blind" sac, meaning that digesta both enters and exits from the upper portion, if the horse eats significant amounts of dry food without sufficient water intake, or if there is a rapid change in diet, the mass can become compacted at the lower end of the caecum, potentially causing colic. Another area is the transverse part of the colon, also known as the pelvic flexure. I am offering this additional diagram (Figure 10) so that this may be seen a little more clearly. [Unfortunately, there seems to be a bit of variation in the equine digestive tract depending upon who is doing the drawing!]

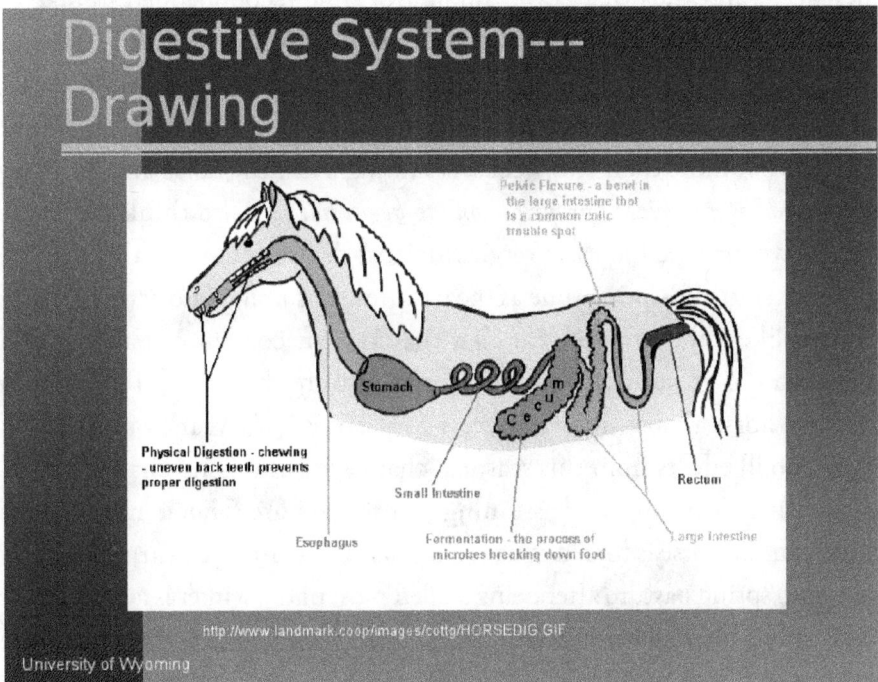

Figure 10: Equine digestive system drawing/Univ of Wyoming
Source: University of Wyoming

The content of the digesta moving from the small intestine into the caecum will mainly consist of undigested fibrous material if the horse is being fed an appropriate raw forage diet. The caecum and the lining of the colon do not produce enzymes; the lining is mucus-secreting only. The digestion taking place in the hindgut primarily relies on microbial fermentation, with only some digestive enzymes being brought down from the small intestine. (Macleod 2007) It is worth noting that while the anatomical design of the large intestine is virtually the same in every horse, the microbial expressions and interactions can be variable depending upon the age and physiological condition of the host. (Williams *et al.* 2001) Furthermore, the microbial populations in the caecum become adaptable to the type of food the horse is allowed to eat; this is the reason it is recommended that any dietary changes be made over a period of time. It is estimated that it takes about three weeks for the populations to adapt to a new feed, and thus that is the amount of time recommended to take to introduce the new feed. (Ohio State University n.d.) [Note: Other sources disagree with this time frame and think it is shorter; regardless the data seems to be empirical only. It is my experience that transitioning can be done in not more than two weeks, assuming a healthy horse and *assuming the "feed" is a species appropriate one to begin with*.] I also think this is the reason we may see increases of grass-related digestive abnormalities in the late winter to mid-spring time as the pastures are coming into active growth. This is likely the time of year that the nutrient content of pastures will undergo the greatest change in a comparatively short period of time. A healthy horse that is allowed access to pasture 24/7 year 'round should suffer no ill effects from this seasonal change (assuming no change in pastures during this time and assuming that the pasture is not a monoculture in which the horse is forced to eat a singular diet). However, turning a horse out onto spring pasture after being stalled most of the winter is at significant risk unless he is given the requisite period of adaptation. And for those horses that have metabolic issues, this can be a challenging time of year, although it should be noted that spring is not the only "danger" time for EMS (Equine Metabolic Syndrome) horses with regard to pasture.

The anaerobic hindgut of the horse is uniquely adapted to maintain a constant neutral or very slightly alkaline pH environment with the fermentative acids being rapidly absorbed through the gut wall and/or neutralized by saliva. This creates an ideal environment for the appropriate microbes, facilitating a symbiotic relationship which gives the horse a steady source of energy derived from the breakdown of fiber, and needed to fuel various metabolic processes. The microbes in the caecum and colon consist of varying stages of bacteria, fungi, and protozoa, with the bacterial stage being the most prevalent one and making the greatest metabolic contribution; the majority of which are gram-negative [at least according to conventional testing procedures]. (van den Berg 2011) Microbial fermentation is defined as "the enzymatic decomposition and utilization of foodstuffs, particularly carbohydrates, by microbes". (Bowen 2010) In carnivores (e.g., dogs and cats) and omnivores (e.g., humans, etc), fermentation is not a significant source of caloric energy; it is, however, in the herbivore. (Bowen 2010) The end products of the fermentation process are volatile fatty acids (VFAs) – primarily propionate, butyrate, and acetate – as well as heat, water, and gas. (Geor 2002) The microbes that are responsible for these end products are not able to fully utilize those products themselves, and so the host animal benefits in energy gain via the absorption of the VFAs into the bloodstream. (van den Berg 2011) Acetate is the principle VFA produced and at least one study (Pethick et al. 1993) has shown that it can be used directly as an energy source by muscle tissue at a rate of up to about 30 percent. (National Research Council 2007) Acetate that is not used to fuel immediate energy needs is likely used for synthesis of long-chain fatty acids, which are either stored for later use or in the case of lactating mares, secreted into the milk. It has been reported (Doreau et al, 1992) that mares consuming high forage rations had higher fat concentrations in their milk than if fed a high-concentration ration (National Research Council 2007) [Remember the "inexplicable" presence of high levels of lipase in the stomach?] Propionate can be used for hepatic glucose synthesis; butyrate has apparently not been studied as much in equines, but it is generally accepted as important in other species. (National Research Council 2007)

The microbial enzymes will also breakdown any undigested proteins that enter the large intestine, although the horse does not benefit from this. Instead, the microbes themselves convert the ammonia that is derived from the protein fermentation back into a form of protein that they can use for their own survival and growth. (Geor 2002) Other products of the microbial fermentation are utilized by the horse, specifically the B-complex vitamins and vitamin K. (Macleod 2007) Any previously undigested sugar (mono- and di-saccharides), starch (non-structural polysaccharides), or soluble fiber (some polysaccharides including some fructans) that reaches the hindgut will be quickly fermented into lactic acid. (Macleod 2007) From a pleomorphic viewpoint, when something is acid forming in the internal terrain, it will in turn morph the microbial population to one that can survive in an acidic environment. While a relatively small and infrequent amount of lactic acid production within the hindgut is likely to not cause long-term adverse consequences, an ongoing situation or a suddenly large amount being produced can have dire consequences, resulting in a situation called subclinical (or hindgut) acidosis. The two most common ways for this to occur are – by feeding a high starch concentrate meal (i.e. one heavy in grains) that is more than the foregut can digest at one time and/or by the horse ingesting too large of an amount of fructans derived from pasture, again greater than the digestive capability of the foregut. (Kentucky Equine Research Staff 2007) Additionally, with sugars, starches, and proteins (as mentioned above) that are fermented instead of digested the horse will forfeit some amount of potential energy to the microbial population. (Alexander 1993) This has significant impact in performance/sport horses that are engaged in energy-demanding activities as the long-term exposure of the large intestinal lining to a low pH environment may negatively affect the absorptive capability of the mucosal lining, thus limiting the potential energy gain. (Kentucky Equine Research Staff 2007) The question is: How much time equates to "long-term"? No one can seem to quantify this and, quite frankly, it can vary to a certain extent from one individual to another. Acidosis can also cause colic situations as well as lead to laminitis. Furthermore, a situation of continual subclinical acidosis can have effects on behavior; stereotypies such as stall weaving and wood chewing have been linked to the discomforts of acidosis in the hindgut. (Kentucky Equine Research Staff 2007) Horses that have undergone extensive colonic resection seem to mount a compensatory response to the attenuating reduction in phosphorus utilization by increasing alkaline phosphatase activity in the caecum and remaining colon. (Hintz and Cymbaluk 1994) This should be kept in mind when analyzing blood work if the particular subject has previously undergone such a surgery.

When we look at ruminant herbivores, we find that their energy utilization is primarily obligate to the absorption of volatile fatty acids in the foregut. Hindgut fermenting herbivores, on the other hand, have the ability for energy gain via enzyme digestion in the foregut prior to the microbial fermentation stage. (van den Berg 2011) There seem to be differing opinions as to which system is more energy efficient (foregut vs. hindgut), but there is no doubt that absorption of VFAs are significant to herbivores regardless of which digestive system they utilize primarily. One interesting aspect of the differences between foregut and hindgut fermenters is that some amount of energy is available in the microbial biomass, meaning that foregut fermenters have the capability of extracting this energy as the biomass leaves the fermentation chamber, whereas in hindgut fermenters this potential energy is lost in the feces. (Alexander 1993)[2] [This is a perfect demonstration of the taxonomical differences between these two species when viewed from within the Goethean classification system; a subject we explore more in behavioral ecology.] What this has been interpreted by some to mean is that comparatively, horses need more highly digestible food than do bovines. In contrast to this there seems to be a well-entrenched theory among many equine authorities and lay people that horses evolved to graze poorer landscapes and not the lush pastures that are so idyllically pictured many times. Alexander's mathematical model seemed to demonstrate the previous - that hindgut fermenters do better on a richer diet when compared to foregut fermenters (horse vs. cow in his model). His model used three different food assumptions: A = very low proportion of cell contents representing mature, low-quality plants; B = plants considerably richer in cell contents such as young leaves; and C = plant stuffs even richer but not some grains and fruits. All versions of his model showed that poor to moderate (A & B) food stuffs were better suited to foregut fermenters, and that hindgut fermentation was optimal only with

---

[2] Note that lagomorphs and other small hindgut fermenters that practice coprophagy with first feces do have the ability to benefit from the energy contained within the microbial biomass.

respect to feeding the richer food (C). (Alexander 1993) Contrast this to the following generalization made by Bell and Janis: where forage quantity is in limited supply, a ruminant digestive system has the advantage; and where forage quality is limited, a caecal (hindgut fermenting) system has the advantage. (Hanley 1982) While this is, in my opinion, by no means an end-all to this discussion, it is interesting to consider when we begin to question and examine why so many horses seemingly can no longer eat grass of any kind without risk of laminitis. I would also ask whether or not the mineral content of any of the feeding models was taken into consideration and what the variances might have been; we will see just how much influence minerals have upon nutrition in that corresponding section.

3.6 Liver and Pancreas

These two organs are considered "accessory organs" relative to the digestive system (Macleod 2007), although they are certainly more than "accessory" to the entire physiology of the horse. Bile produced by the liver is necessary for fat digestion and neutralization of the contents in the small intestine. As mentioned before, the pancreas produces digestive enzymes and pancreatic juices, also necessary for digestion and neutralization. (Macleod 2007) The liver functions significantly in the processing of nutrients after absorption, which also means that the liver will function significantly in the processing of any toxins that may be in the feed, whether from naturally occurring sources (such as toxic plants) or put there with intention (such as chemicals in processed feed). The absorbed nutrients are carried via the hepatic portal vein from the gut directly to the liver, with one exception – fats. The metabolic products of dietary fat digestion are released into the lymphatic system where they are then released gradually into the blood. Protein carriers are required to transport fats from the gut, which the liver produces.

3.7   SUMMARY OF PHYSIOLOGY

With regard to their digestive system, we can conventionally classify animals by one of two ways (or both): food source or stomach type. Horses, classified by food source, are herbivores...meaning they are primarily plant eaters. In order to digest the tough fibrous material found in plant cell walls, there must be some kind of fermentation process in the digestive tract. Therefore, if we classify horses by stomach type, they are known as hindgut fermenters; meaning their fermentation capability is primarily located post-gastric or after the stomach. Compare this to cattle (a ruminant) whose fermentation capability is located pre-gastric. In the horse, the majority of the microbial fermentation occurs in the colon (as opposed to the caecum – roughly 38% compared to 15%, colon vs. caecum). There are generally two classes of herbivores: ruminating and non-ruminating, the latter having a single-chamber stomach as opposed to the multi-chamber stomach of ruminants. Horses, therefore, are monogastric herbivores. The stomach and small intestine in the horse is comparatively similar to other monogastric species; it is the sheer size of the horse's hindgut that is rather remarkable among monogastric herbivores.

A horse, like any other animal, has requirements for energy, protein, vitamins, and minerals. Energy is derived when food is broken down into its constituent parts and thus digested and absorbed. In the gastric part of the horse's digestive system, the glandular portion of the stomach secretes acid, mucous, and pepsinogen; little actual digestion takes place here, the digesta is mainly being prepared for entry into the small intestine. Major digestion of most non-structural carbohydrates occurs in the small intestine through a hydrolytic process that breaks carbohydrates down into simple sugars.

While enzyme digestion is considered "true" digestion, the microbial fermentation that primarily takes place in the horse's hindgut should not be taken lightly with regard to the contribution it has toward the nutrient and energy requirements of the horse, or any animal that has this capability. One of the important aspects of microbial fermentation is the retention time, defined as the time the plant material is in contact with the microbes, thus dictating the extent of digestion. While longer retention time certainly results in more complete digestion (and thus more energy), there is an upper limit. The by-products of microbial fermentation are volatile fatty acids (VFAs); however, if the retention time is excessive, the VFAs themselves will be degraded, thus depriving the horse of energy.

Even though much progress has been made in recent years, we still do not have a complete understanding about the biology of the horse's digestive system. Many if not most studies of the aspects of a horse's nutritional requirements have been performed in vitro (in the laboratory). While this certainly has some value, it can be difficult at best many times to extrapolate those results back to the biology of the intact organism. This is the difference between viewing something from a biochemical aspect versus a biophysical aspect. If at all possible without causing harm to the subject, studies performed in vivo render much more valuable information. We may also glean some valuable knowledge by studying the evolutionary nutritional basis for food selection (for ungulates in particular) which requires an in-depth understanding of the physiological aspects of the digestive anatomy in the particular species.

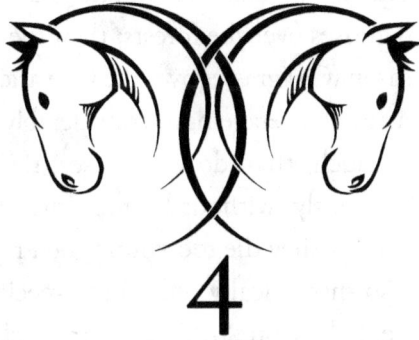

4
BASIC NUTRIENT REQUIREMENTS

T HE ANCESTRAL HORSE began as a browser, then about 17 - 20 million years ago (the latter part of the early Miocene period), a watershed occurred in the development of what would eventually lead to our modern horse. He began moving out of the forest and swampy areas onto the plains as the climate changed to favor conditions for grasslands over dense forests. Paleontologists have been able to determine this occurrence based upon the analysis that grasses are typically much more abrasive than are the leaves of trees and shrubs, which reflected in a distinct change in the wear of the dentition found in fossil records. (Olsen 2003) (p 25) The horse's ancestral tree branched significantly after this with the different species being split between those that had long teeth and those that retained the shorter ones of previous evolutionary periods; this ensuing period also saw the emergence of a new species of horse that had very long teeth (likely comparable to what we see in modern horse today). This diversity continued until about 6 million years ago when there was a suddenly large extinction pulse resulting in a drastic loss of total diversity, leaving only those horses with the very longest teeth. The conventional theories have suggested that it was the loss of forestation alone that triggered this extinction. Yet, that doesn't make sense if the various horse species were already developing dentition in the form of longer teeth that were more adapted to grazing grasses than browsing. What paleobiologist Steven Stanley discovered was that the climate change initially began to favor temperate (C3) grasses over the forests; then the climate shifted into one favoring warm season (C4) grasses over the C3 varieties. The distinction of this is that C4 grasses on average have considerably more silica content (about three times as much) than do C3 grasses, thus causing advanced wear of the teeth. Obviously, without human intervention, if the horse cannot eat, then he dies; if they die too young then reproductive viability is lost in the species, so theoretically only those species with very longest of teeth would survive. (Clarkson 2010) And this is what we have today… horses that are very well adapted to grazing, with some limited preference at certain times of the year for browsing depending upon what is available.

What is interesting to consider in the pre-domestication times of the horse is that he obviously had the ability to "rank potential food items according to their net value". (Hanley 1982) Plants are highly variable, with variations occurring not just intra-, but inter-species; diurnally; seasonally; etc. The horse would obviously have to have some type of innate ability to keep track of these changing nutritional values of his food source.

Food (and that includes water) is required to nourish all living beings; that is for growth, repair, and to fuel all the energy systems in the body. From a biophysical viewpoint, there is a huge difference between a diet that nourishes the body and one that sustains the bodily functions (the biochemical view). In the following sub-chapters we will cover the six basic nutrients that all animals require. Some animals will require more of one nutrient than others; for instance, carnivores require a significant amount of protein. Herbivores, on the other hand, require only a fairly steady and relatively low amount of protein but require a significant amount of carbohydrates in various forms, including fiber.

In the following sections we will look more closely at the various nutrient requirements of the horse. Sources for the following include: Batmanghelidj 1995, Hoffman 2003, Johnson and Duberstein 2010, Kentucky Performance Products Staff 2012, National Research Council 2007, Macleod 2007, Pagan 1998a, the author's own knowledge gleaned from years of study and observation, and those references specifically noted.

4.1 WATER

All life requires water to function and the necessity of it for horses should be obvious as a normal, healthy horse will consume 5-15 gallons of water per day, and even more, depending upon factors such as temperature, humidity, level of exercise, etc. The quality of water, however, can have a significant impact upon health. Horses, like many species can survive longer without food than without water. Water is used to propel food through the gastro-intestinal tract; along with enzymes, it hydrolyzes nutrients for transport throughout the body; it acts as a vehicle to also transport excesses and wastes so they can be excreted; it is a medium for all metabolic processes; and can play a significant role in regulating the body temperature. The balance of fluids in the body is controlled by hormones, and as in many species, the kidneys function to maintain the overall balance of bodily fluids.

Horses obtain water from not just direct drinking but also in food and from daily metabolic processes. It is always best to allow the horse free access to water at all times so they can self-regulate their intake depending upon their feed intake as well as other internal processes occurring. Spring grasses will typically have as much as 80% water content; on the other hand, regular (non-fermented) hay is usually about 10% in moisture content. Fermented hay (a.k.a. haylage) is typically about 55% moisture content (Steve Rader, Pres. and CEO, Chaffhaye, via email 03/14/12). Lack of sufficient water can range from mild dehydration to death; insufficient water intake can cause intestinal impaction, especially when being fed concentrates or dry hay.

Fat contains considerably less water than does lean muscle tissue. (Winona State University 2000) This becomes significant in those horses that have excess fat deposits, a symptom that we have associated with insulin resistance, also known as Equine Metabolic Syndrome (EMS). There will be an associated state of chronic dehydration in these horses, so it becomes even more important to allow free access to water, as well as making sure the horse is actually drinking. Chronic dehydration is different than acute dehydration; it is not something you can determine via a "pinch test" or capillary refill rate. The current scientific paradigm regards solutes as regulators and water only as a solvent and a means of transport within the body. In other words, science, for the biggest part does not look upon water as a regulator of body functions (other than thermoregulation), including the regulation of water intake itself. This has led to the often times erroneous assumption that we can identify one particular "substance" as the cause of a particular disease, and it then looks upon clinical dehydration as a resulting symptom of some underlying "disease". In addition to what is listed above, some of the other properties of water include: 1) the "hydroelectric energy" (Batmanghelidj 1995) that is converted and stored in the form of ATP and GTP, vital substances used in energy transfer within the body; and 2) the facilitation of the metabolism of proteins and enzymes at cell receptor points in solutions of lower viscosity (state of hydration). In states of chronic dehydration (solutions of higher viscosity), there has potentially been much damage at the cellular level, and the body has already begun a system of rationing and re-distribution. In humans, according to Dr. Batmanghelidj, we can see these results in the clinical symptoms of ulcers, high blood pressure, and heart "disease, to name just a few. In the case of humans, the thirst reaction (from dry mouth) is one of the last symptoms of chronic dehydration. With horses in a native setting, this should never become a problem (assuming a supply of water is available) as their instincts remain intact. The issue with domestication is whether or not the horse's instinctual behavior patterns remain completely intact or have they been altered to some degree. I have not yet come across studies of this nature to much extent, but as the field of equine welfare advances, these issues are likely to be looked into more in depth (including by this author). I offer the following quote via group email May 29, 2012, (with permission) from Andy Beck, equine ethologist:

> "One line from one of the previous posts caught my eye: Horses have physically adapted to the inadequate housing and keeping arrangement of most domestic settings.............. and I feel strongly that this isn't true. The balance of everything I've seen over the last twenty years

has convinced me that we have not changed horses very much at all, and that any changes we have made are very small. Management that ignores the nature of the animal and its needs still causes massive problems, just as it has always done. And this is not only true of horses but equally true of other domesticated animals (yep, pigs need lots of movement too – who would have thought it?) as much as it is true for us. Human bodies that don't get enough exercise age faster get ill more often and deteriorate more rapidly. Neither our animals nor us have adapted to 'modern' life – and in many cases it is killing both them and us by degrees – as well as making us look high and low for therapy."

I agree that horses have certainly not "adapted to…inadequate…domestic settings" with respect to overall welfare requirement, but I also think these very same domestic settings can alter their innate sensory mechanisms.

While there are many issues surrounding the quality of water, for the sake of brevity I will briefly address one of the primary concerns for those who are on municipal water supplies and that is the fluoridation of the water supply. Although there is still much controversy surrounding this issue with heated debate on both sides, in my professional opinion, the science now stands behind the toxicity of added fluoride to water supplies – there have been way too many studies that show this to ignore it any longer - and especially when you consider the sheer quantity that horses consume. Visit http://www.youtube.com/watch?v=4WeEj-dUaDIk to watch a video that documents how the fluoridation of the municipal water supply in

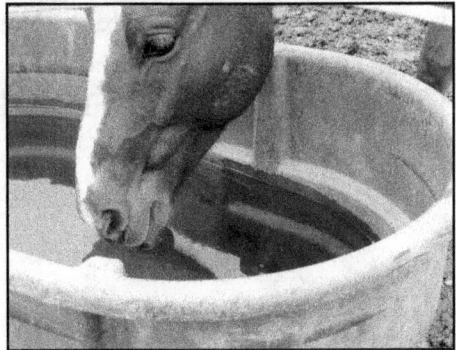

Figure 11: Horse drinking water
Shutterstock.com image # 725714; © Sarah Cates

Pagosa Springs, CO caused multiple pathological conditions – and death – in horses and dogs:

Further documentation on fluoride poisoning in horses can be found at http://www.fluorideresearch.org/391/files/3913-10.pdf

The other issues with water quality involve the mineral content, especially for those on wells, and which can vary considerably from one region to another as well as from one locality to another. If one is experiencing inexplicable clinical issues with their horses, getting the water tested may be a step toward diagnosis.

Another aspect of water quality involves something that is still controversial especially among those that are not open to intangible aspects of things. Much of science still demands tangible results from studies and does not have the capability to deal with the 'unseen"; however quantum physics is showing us pathways we never before thought possible. I will just briefly mention this and the student/reader can research this further and come to your own conclusions. As we all know, water does not naturally flow in straight lines – it meanders, it rolls, it cascades, it falls...the water in a river that has not been mechanically altered, never flows in a straight line. And, we pipe in our drinking water in straight pipes (allowing for an elbow here and there). Some say that forcing water through a straight path voids the energy and electric potential of the water. Attaching a vortex device to your water supply can restore the energetic and electrical potential of the water. Yet others avow the healing properties of magnetizing the water or sending it through "special" filters. There is a "caveat emptor" with any of these devices – do your research first!

4.2 Carbohydrates

When it comes to equine nutrition, many people equate carbohydrates[3] with only the type of food that is digestible by enzymes in the foregut of the horse – i.e. 'non-structural carbs', although even this is not correct as we will see. You may hear people say "I need a 'low-carb' diet for my overweight horse." If one were to feed a true 'low-carb' diet, it would also equate to a low amount of fiber! To say that the subject of carbohydrates in equine nutrition can be confusing is an understatement. Even those employed in the equine nutrition industry are not consistent among themselves with respect to nomenclature, although I feel at a loss to offer a plausible explanation for this as there is no real reason why it should be this way. Therefore, I will attempt to stay within the boundaries of established science when discussing carbohydrates while giving the student/reader reference to common terms used equatively, and at the same time, hopefully, not making this more boring than necessary. Please keep in mind this discussion is relative to equine nutrition only, not any other species.

The equine digestive physiology regarding carbohydrates can be divided into two very broad groups – those that can be hydrolyzed in the foregut (primarily small intestine with some hydrolyzation via stomach acid) and those that are fermented in the hindgut into VFAs. This does not, however, take into consideration that there is some fermentative capability within the foregut (as discussed in the previous chapter), although there is little to no energy gain from it, at least as yet determined. The location of carbohydrate digestion is determined by the link between the glucose units: beta bonds cannot be broken by digestive enzymes, thus the resistant

---

[3] A system of nutrient component classification should correlate to analytical techniques if it is to be of any real use in actual implementation; this book and course will attempt to follow those guidelines when they exist. It will, however, deviate via explanation when it would seem to facilitate learning. This mostly affects carbohydrates and fiber. It should be understood that most analytical techniques currently being used for equine nutrition were adapted (or simply ported over in use) from those designed for ruminant type digestive systems; to my knowledge there is no set of nutrient analyzes that were formulated specifically with the horse's digestive system in mind. One of the primary drawbacks, in this author's opinion at least, occurs when one is trying to determine the amount of energy generated by a particular food in one or the other type of digestion (hydrolysis vs fermentation), given the fact that ruminant fermentation is considerably different than equine fermentation.

Additionally, there are no absolutes when it comes to the function of individual organisms and so any analytical techniques should be used as guidelines only.

starches and structural and soluble components of fiber flow to the hindgut where microbial fermentation can achieve this; alpha bonds are digestible by enzymes and so the food components containing non-resistant starches and the sugars are hydrolyzed in the small intestine.

In 2001, Hoffman et al. devised a partitioning system for equine feeds that resulted in the following three basic categories. Methods for analyzing all of these fractions, however, are not readily available. (National Research Council 2007):

▶ Hydrolyzable carbohydrates (CHO-H) which are the simple sugars and non-resistant starches, including some (non-fructan) oligo-saccharides; while there may be some relatively small amount of fermentation in the stomach, the primary characteristic is that they can be degraded quickly down to monosaccharides in the small intestine, resulting in a quickly available source of energy

▶ Rapidly fermentable carbohydrates (CHO-FR) which are readily available for microbial fermentation in the hindgut; they include the pectins, fructans, and the oligosaccharides not digested in the foregut, as well as resistant starch and some hemicellulose – i.e., primarily the polysaccharides that have a larger degree of solubility

▶ Slowly fermentable carbohydrates (CHO-FS) include the structural carbohydrates such as cellulose and hemicellulose – i.e., the non-sol-uble polysaccharides that result primarily in acetate production in the hindgut

    ▼ Note: resistant starches are basically those that resist enzyme degradation and thus are typically digested in the hindgut via microbial fermentation; non-resistant starches are those that can be digested by enzymes. Some equine nutritionists will clas-sify as resistant starches those components that escape foregut hydrolyzation and flow to fermentation in the hindgut simply due to an overfeeding situation. I disagree with this assessment as it ignores the accepted science and applies a label that is solely generated by mismanagement of feeding. It does not change the structure of the carbohydrate.

Carbohydrates are the principle source of energy for a horse, providing fuel for daily metabolic processes as well as additional energy as needed for certain levels of activity. Energy value is derived from glucose absorption prececal plus carbohydrates that are fermented into VFAs in the hindgut. The horse is especially adapted for "time-release" glucose absorption - meaning, from natural sources over the diurnal period, and not processed feeds fed in a couple of large meals. The breakdown of the simple sugars and starches in the foregut supplies this glucose which is then absorbed through the small intestine, becoming immediately available for energy needs via the bloodstream. And like humans, the horse stores excess glucose in the form of glycogen in muscle tissue and the liver for later use.

Many nutritional fibers are classified as carbohydrates, although some are not (such as lignin). Although some people may think of fiber as dietary "filler", given the fact that the horse's digestive tract is designed to process high levels of fiber, it is an extremely important carbohydrate in equine nutrition. Furthermore, all herbivores need a certain amount of non-digestible fiber for gastrointestinal motility.

Chemically, carbohydrates (CHO) contain carbon combined with hydrogen and oxygen, usually in the same ratio as in water. Their basic repeating unit is the monosaccharide, and they can be categorized by what is known as degree of polymerization (DP). All carbohydrates are saccharides. Polymerization is a chemical reaction, in which two or more molecules combine to form larger molecules which contain "chains", or repeating structural units of the original molecule; in nature under ordinary conditions, enzymes are the catalysts that carry out this process, forming proteins, nucleic acids, and carbohydrate polymers. (Merriam-Webster. com dictionary) It is the different bonds linking these various chains that determine where and how they can be digested – or even if they can be digested (see alpha and beta bonds above). Therefore the DP signifies the number of monosaccharide units in a carbohydrate chain.

Monosaccharides and disaccharides (one and two saccharide molecules, respectively) are what we commonly refer to as the "sugars" in a horse's diet. The monosaccharides are the simplest molecular carbohydrate unit and cannot be digestively broken down further. We can refer to monosaccharides as the building blocks for fuel (energy) and nucleic acids; they are either aldehydes or ketones. Monosaccharides of importance in equine nutrition are:

▶ Glucose - blood sugar

▶ Fructose – "fruit" sugar (is polymerized to make fructans which are found in forages)

▶ Galactose - found in hemicellulose

▶ Mannose - found in hemicellulose

▶ Arabinose - found in hemicellulose

▶ Xylose - found in hemicellulose

Free monosaccharides occur in low concentrations in plants – the only ones appearing free in nature are glucose and fructose. Glucose is the immediate product of photosynthesis in plants. Monosaccharides are the only form of carbohydrate that can be absorbed via the small intestine, which is done by digestive and plant enzymes.[4]

Disaccharides that are important to the horse are:

▶ Lactose – composed of glucose & galactose; a.k.a. milk sugar; is important in nursing foals

▶ Maltose – consists of two glucose units; produced in the GI tract by the action of amylase on starch; may be further broken down into glucose

Oligosaccharides can present a bit of a conundrum within equine nutrition and some nutritionists will simply ignore them as a separate DP class, some calling them simple sugars (specifically disaccharides) while others label them as polysaccharides. The Nutrient Requirements of Horses, 6th Ed., classifies oligosaccharides as having a DP of 3-10, thus falling in between the simple

---

[4] This author has not come across any references specific to equine nutrition science that recognizes the function of plant enzymes, although human nutrition contains a number of scientific references. It is my position that this is an underexplored – or even ignored - area of equine nutrition and I will continue to at least give it mention.

sugars and the polysaccharides. Even though they are non-structural, oligosaccharides are generally resistant to hydrolysis by mammalian digestive enzymes, being readily fermentable by enteric bacteria. (Note that enteric in this sense is not restricted to the small intestine and in this case probably refers more to the large intestine.) Oligosaccharides can fall in both the CHO-H and CHO-FR categories depending upon what type they are. The purpose of at least some oligosaccharides may be that of a "prebiotic". Prebiotics can be defined as non-digestible food components that can have beneficial effects on the host by selectively stimulating certain bacteria. Some of the oligosaccharides of importance to the horse are:

▸ Raffinose – a trisaccharide consisting of galactose, fructose, and glucose; found in legumes and sugar beets

▸ Stachyose – a tetrasaccharide consisting of two galactose, one glucose, and one fructose units; it can be found in plants including soybean

▸ Maltotriose – a trisaccharide consisting of three glucose molecules

▸ Fructooligosaccharide (FOS) – composed of short chains of fructose and is one type of fructan of significance in equine nutrition (a.k.a. oligofructan); can also be known as a prebiotic; they are found in various pasture plants (including those plants some people call "weeds")

Mono-, di-, and oligosaccharides are all soluble carbohydrates. Mono- and disaccharides as well as some of the oligosaccharides (such as maltotriose) are primarily digested via hydrolysis in the small intestine and are therefore included the CHO-H category. Raffinose, stachyose, and FOS, on the other hand, are only available for microbial fermentation in the hindgut; they are in the CHO-FR category.

Polysaccharides are a significantly large group of carbohydrates, defined as having greater than 10 monosaccharide units. They can be either non-structural – including polysaccharide fructans; soluble fiber; or structural. Soluble fiber and structural polysaccharides – as well as non-carbohydrate fiber - will be discussed below under the category of Fiber, as this is a complex and many times misunderstood, albeit very significant, portion of a horse's diet. The non-structural carbohydrates, or NSC, fraction of total carbohydrates is a broader fraction than just the non-structural polysaccharides; thus the NSC value includes sugars and starches as well as fructan. Nonstructural carbohydrates are easily digested by the horse's own digestive tract, primarily in the small intestine. These sugars and starches are primarily found in grains (i.e. corn, oats, barley, etc.) and provide a more concentrated form of energy to the horse than do structural carbohydrates (hence the term "concentrates" is often used when referring to grains and grain mixtures). Lower amounts of varying degree are found in pasture plants.

All starches are non-structural polysaccharides and consist of two forms: 1) amylose has a linear unbranched chain of glucose units and 2) amylopectin is a multi-branched glucose chain. According to many references, amylase (the enzyme that digests starches) is found in relatively low quantities in the horse's saliva and/or small intestine suggesting a distinct limitation in starch digestion; however the Nutrient Requirements of Horses, 6th Ed., makes reference to the "abundance of amylase in the digestive secretions" (p38), although unfortunately no source for this statement is given. The comparisons in determining this "deficit" (if it does indeed exist) seem to be with either humans or pigs, and it is not clear as to how this determination was made; i.e., what type of feed (natural or processed) was used to generate amylase for measurement in the analysis. Regardless, none of the references take into consideration the amylase inherent in plants. Once again, we have to look at the physiology of the horse's digestive tract that tells us he is designed to ingest small amounts of starch on a frequent basis from natural forages, not in a couple of starch-heavy processed meals per day which lack the inherent food enzymes. The relatively fast passage rate of digesta through the foregut is also indicative of the horse requiring small amounts of starches at any given time. It is this author's opinion there is completely sufficient total amylase available for starch digestion when fed a species appropriate diet, and that this cannot therefore be deemed a physiological "deficiency". When starch is digested in the foregut, it is done so by hydrolyzation (enzyme activity) with the end product being glucose, which as we have seen, the horse is very capable of utilizing. When starch passes to the hindgut it becomes food for starch loving bacteria, whose end products are propionic acid and large amounts of lactic acid. Lactic acid can certainly be used as a source of energy without problems – in amounts that do not exceed the body's metabolic capabilities; this capability can vary drastically from one individual to another depending upon many factors. Exceeding this capability produces a build-up of acid in the hindgut. In any equine diet, the bulk of starch should be digested in the foregut.

The non-structural polysaccharides that are important in equine nutrition consist primarily of starches and polysaccharide fructans. Some fructans (those that are not oligosaccharides) are considered polysaccharides as they have greater than 10 monosaccharide units however they have a lower DP than most other polysaccharides. Polysaccharide fructans are technically soluble fiber, but they are handled as a non-structural carbohydrate in equine feed analyzes. As opposed to starches, which are made up of glucose chains, all fructans are made up of fructose chains. Fructan was originally found in 1804 in a hot water extract of the plant Inula helenium, later known as 'inulin'. (Taiz and Zeiger 2010) Inulin is a polysaccharide fructan of importance in equine nutrition. Both starches and fructans are referred to as "reserve carbohydrates" with respect to plant physiology.[5] Starches fall into the CHO-H category, being available for foregut

---

[5] Plants have the ability to "fix" atmospheric carbon dioxide during periods of photosynthesis (the presence of light), which results in the production of simple sugars (aka carbohydrates). When these sugars (carbohydrates) are produced in excess of the current energy needs, they are stored in the plants cells for later use as needed. This is a survival mechanism and can happen during periods of low growth, such as in winter, as well as periods of drought, etc. This reserve is typically stored in warm season (C4) pasture plants and legumes as starch within the leaves and is self-limiting. However, the reserves in cool season (C3) pasture grasses are stored as fructans; furthermore they are stored in the stems of the plants and appear to have no self-limiting mechanism, resulting in potentially high concentrations diurnally as well as seasonally. While research can give us the "normal" sequence of variations, it should be borne in mind that microclimate as well as various environmental factors can affect these "norms" to a wide range of degrees. It is therefore important to understand the underlying principles of carbohydrate production and storage in pasture plants and apply those principles to your own individual environment. Fructans are oligo- and polyfructose molecules that function as non-structural (soluble) carbohydrates. Some researchers believe that fructans are not digestible by mammalian enzymes, and so it is assumed that horses have this very limited capability to digest this type of sugar with much of the fructans passing relatively intact to the hindgut. However both starch (from C4 grasses) as well as fructans (from C3 grasses) can wreak havoc in the hindgut if there is a large influx of either (or both). It is believed that the appearance of a large amount of starch or fructans in the hindgut will trigger the activity of certain bacteria that produce lactic acid (amylolytic and saccharolytic bacteria), thus having the potential to suddenly and drastically lower the pH of the hindgut when it is designed to maintain a neutral pH. This can have far-reaching effects; not the least of which is a high state of acidosis and can trigger acute laminitis. If you add chronic insulin resistance to this mix, then you have a formula for chronic laminitis. And, of course, the chronic insulin resistance can be triggered by an ongoing influx of more starches and/or fructans than the horse is designed to process. (Longland and Byrd 2006)

hydrolyzation. All fructans, on the other hand, are digested in the hindgut via microbial fermentation and are part of the CHO-FR category.

4.3 FIBER

All forages consist of two primary components – cell walls and cell contents. The cell contents contain the soluble and hydrolyzable fractions of the plant - all the starches, sugars, lipids, organic acids, soluble ash, and most of the protein. The cell wall contains the resistant, structural carbohydrate fractions – cellulose, hemicellulose, pectin, gums and mucilages; as well as lignin, which is not a carbohydrate. We can determine the nutritive value of the plant by two factors: the fiber content, which is composed of the cell wall; and the fiber quality, which represents the degree of lignification. In other words, the amount of lignin depends upon the maturity of the plant and will thus largely affect the degree to which fiber can be digested. (Pagan 2009)[6] In this section, we will be concerned with the fibrous cell wall fractions.

Fibers vary in solubility. Legumes in general tend to have higher solubility than do grasses. When we talk about solubility of carbohydrates in horse feed (including forages), we are referring to the component's ability to dissolve in water, which affects digestibility. The soluble fibers include pectin, gums and mucilages, and some hemicellulose. Pectin is composed of chains of galacturonic acid residues as well as the sugars arabinose and galactose. It is a type of fiber that is soluble and forms a gel in the presence of water. Pectin is very digestible in the hindgut and can be found in high quantities in sugar beets and apples. Gums contain galactose, glucuronic

---

[6] Digestibility of cut forages are indirectly measured by a test called Acid Detergent Fiber content, or ADF, and determines the amount of cellulose and lignin in the hay. The more mature the hay, the higher the levels of cellulose and lignin, and the less the digestibility of the hay (i.e., more "stemmy" hay). Neutral detergent fiber (NDF) is a measure of the cell wall content, which increases as the plant matures; it is an indirect measure of the palatability of a forage, or how readily it is consumed [although this can be somewhat subjective from one individual horse to another]. Therefore, more desirable horse hays will have both low ADF and NDF measures. Maturity is related to the stage when hay is cut and not to the time of year of the cutting. (Russell and Johnson 2007) It should be noted, however, that one does NOT want to feed 100% digestible fiber on a continual basis, else risk stagnation of the digestive tract that can lead to GI disorders such as enteritis or colic. (Kentucky Equine Research Staff 2011a)

acid and other monosaccharides; mucilages contain galactose, mannose and other monosaccharides. They are also soluble and form a gel-like consistency in the presence of water. Gums and mucilages are completely digestible in the large intestine. Seaweed is a type of mucilage that is digestible in the horse's hindgut. (Macleod 2007) Soluble fibers fall into the CHO-FR classification.

Cellulose and hemicellulose are considered structural fiber polysaccharides. Cellulose is not water soluble and its degradation in the hindgut varies but is typically low. It is composed of linked polymers of glucose. Hemicellulose can vary in solubility as well as its fermentative ability in the hindgut. It consists of several different sugars: arabinose, xylose, glucose, fucose (another monosaccharide not previously mentioned), mannose, and galactose. Cellulose and hemicellulose are typically found in close association, but hemicellulose is not a precursor to cellulose. The content of cellulose and hemicellulose in pasture grasses will increase with maturity. (Macleod 2007) Cellulose and hemicellulose are classified as CHO-FS. They are also classified as SC, or structural carbohydrates.

Lignin is another form of structural, but non-soluble, fiber found in mature plants, especially the stems, that cannot be digested by either direct digestive enzyme action or by microbial fermentation action in the hindgut and thus will pass in the manure; it is not classified as a carbohydrate. (Macleod 2007)

Dietary fiber is sometimes (if not often) referred to as a non-starch polysaccharide (NSP), but there are some sources (including Macleod) that seem to not be in favor of this as NSP also includes (some) fructans. Combining fiber into one classification such as this ignores the fact that some fibers are rapidly fermented while others are slowly fermented. Rapidly fermentable CHO can yield lactic acid; therefore if too much (as in the case of fructan) passes to the hindgut with resulting lactic acid increase, this can cause a cascade of problems not the least of which may result in laminitis. Of course, the definition of "how much is too much" can vary from one individual to another depending upon a whole host of co-factors. Slowly fermentable carbohydrates, on the other hand typically do not cause metabolic issues, yielding mostly acetate and butyrate; but they also may not supply enough energy for our modern "use" of horses, especially those used intensively in performance such as racing and eventing.

In summary, we can characterize forages by their high dietary fiber content being primarily composed of structural carbohydrates (SC) found in the plant wall and the varying amounts of lignin (depending upon the maturity of the plant). Non-structural carbohydrates (NSC) which represent the cell contents including the simple sugars and storage carbohydrates such as starch and fructan are also found in forages. These two values together constitute the main energy-yielding fractions of forage. Starch is digested to glucose by the endogenous enzymes found in the small intestine (as well as food based enzymes); those resulting sugars along with any free sugars will metabolize across the small intestine yielding ATP (adenosine triphosphate). The amount of starch digested in the foregut will be dependent upon the quantity, botanical origin, the co-feeds, the quantity of amylolytic enzymes, as well as any physiological variations of particular horses. Mammals do not have gut enzymes that can digest fructans; they are however degradable by lactic acid producing bacteria. Therefore, the SC components as well as fructans pass to the hindgut where they are converted to VFAs by the resident microbes which in turn yield ATP (energy). (National Research Council 2007), p 141)

Methods exist for measuring some but not all carbohydrate fractions in animal feeds (including grass and hay). Due to the difficulty in measuring some components, various partitioning systems have been devised over the years. The one developed by Van Soest in the late 1960's is still today the most common one used, although others are developing newer or revised ones (as stated above with Hoffman et al.). Most analytical methods were devised for ruminants, not horses.

4.4 LIPIDS (FATS & OILS)

Dietary fats can provide energy as well as supply essential fatty acids (EFAs) and act as a carrier for fat-soluble vitamins (A, D, E, and K). Enzymes (primarily the lipases) are necessary to break fats down into fatty acids. Fat digestion in the horse occurs in the small intestine. Omega 3 and omega 6 fatty acids are termed "essential" in the diet as most mammals cannot synthesize these; omega 9 can typically be synthesized so long as there are sufficient amounts of omega 3 in the diet. In humans, an inability to digest and assimilate fats can lead to disorders of the skin and hair. (Loomis 2007) The requirements of fat in the horse's diet relates to essential fatty acids. (Hallebeek and A.C. Beynen 2002) Deficiencies have not been reported and general EFA requirements in the horse have not been established, although it is suggested that a dietary minimum for linoleic acid (omega 6) is 0.5 percent of dry matter (DM). (National Research Council 2007) It has been clinically demonstrated that omega 3 fatty acids have the same beneficial effects in horses as they do in humans. It should be noted that pastures typically contain higher omega-3 levels than omega-6, and that grains are the opposite, containing higher omega-6 EFAs than omega-3s. In generalized terms, omega-3s are anti-inflammatory, and omega-6s are pro-inflammatory. There is still debate in the human sector as to what ratio is ideal, but it is generally accepted that the modern human diet contains far too many omega-6s in relation to omega-3s; it seems this same trend has carried over to feeding our horses.

Biochemically, fats and oils belong to the large group of compounds known as lipids; which in turn are either hydrophobic (water-repelling) or amphiphilic (meaning both water-loving and fat-loving simultaneously – Wikipedia 06/28/12) and can be either glycerol or nonglycerol based. Those that are glycerol based include glycolipids, phospholipids, and triglycerides; nonglycerol based lipids include cholesterol and its fatty acid esters. (National Research Council 2007) All fats and oils are triglyceride molecules based on glycerol and formed by the reaction with fatty acids (triglycerides are also called triacylglycerols). In generalized terms (and there can be exceptions) – fats are solid at room temperature, are derived from animal sources, and are saturated; oils are liquid at room temperature, come from non-animal sources (i.e. plants), and are non-saturated. (Eggling and Clackamas Community College 2001, 2003) However, the term "dietary fat" tends to be used within equine nutrition to mean both fats and oils, primarily the latter. Glucose can be generated from glycerol (as well as other non-carbohydrate sources such as protein/amino acids, lactate, and others) through a process known as gluconeogenesis that primarily takes place in the liver and to a lesser extent, in the kidneys. It can occur during periods of fasting, starvation, low carbohydrate diets, or intense exercise and is one of two mechanisms by which animals (including humans) use to prevent hypoglycemia, i.e. low blood sugar; the other mechanism is through the degradation of glycogen (glycogenolysis).

We saw above that excess glucose is stored as glycogen for future energy needs. Additionally, when glycogen sites are full, glucose and amino acids are used to synthesize lipids, meaning that glycogen and adipose tissue both are used for long-term energy storage needs. Fat – or adipose – tissue is found in two different forms in mammals…white and brown fat. White adipose tissue serves three functions – 1) a reservoir for storing excess energy; 2) cushioning and protecting various body organs from damage; and 3) thermoregulation via insulation (i.e the retention of heat in the body when exposed to cold). (Albright and Stern J.S 1998), (Stover 2003) The function of brown fat is to generate heat by the transfer of energy from food to heat. Put simply, the differences between the two with regard to energy are that white fat stores energy and brown fat dissipates energy. (Lowell and Flier 1997) Exposure to cold can trigger the activation of brown fat. In most cells, the mitochondria convert glucose and fat into ATP, the energy currency which the body uses. However, brown fat contains an "uncoupling" protein that diverts energy away from ATP synthesis, instead favoring heat production. This process is tightly regulated by signaling from the sympathetic nervous system. Animals that are adapted to the cold display an increased production of heat from brown fat. (Stover 2003) (This is yet another reason to not blanket a healthy horse in the winter time.)

Brown fat has been getting a lot of attention in human research in recent years as leading to a possible way to "treat" obesity and the corresponding complications of glucose intolerance and diabetes. Researchers in the laboratory of Bruce Spiegelman, PhD, of the Dana-Farber Cancer Institute in Boston, MA, reported the discovery of a "new" hormone released by muscle that converts white fat deposits into thermogenic brown fat; they called this hormone irisin. (Laidman 2012) Apparently irisin levels rise with exercise, and perhaps some other as yet unknown factors. The current reports indicate that the hormone can improve glucose tolerance as well as increase insulin production, thus helping to prevent full blown Type II diabetes in humans. Given the implications of insulin in laminitis, I think it quite prudent to conduct considerable more research before assuming that horses can also benefit from any resulting "treatments" (such as intra-muscular injections of irisin) that may be derived from research in the human sector. Insulin resistance in horses does not necessarily follow the same metabolic pathways that diabetes or even pre-diabetes in humans does (a subject beyond the scope of this book).

Nevertheless, dietary fat (oils, to be more precise) has been getting some attention in the equine performance sector in recent years as a partial substitute for carbohydrates in the overall total diet. With the increasing energy demands of performance horses, people began feeding more carbohydrates in the form of concentrates, with the resulting onslaught of metabolic and physiological issues. Thus, the perceived advantages of replacing some of the CHO load with fat. Fat storage requires less water and less overall mass than does carbohydrate storage. (Albright and Stern J.S 1998) Horses on a natural "raw" diet will get sufficient levels of alpha-linoleic acid (omega-3 EFA); a typical pasture diet will contain 3% - 4%. In a natural habitat, during certain times of the year, grasses will produce seed (typically late summer/early fall) and horses have been observed eating seed heads during these times; presumably increasing some amount of fat storage for colder months as energy reserves as well as insulation. This obviously has been completely sufficient for the evolutionary requirements of the horse. In humans, a normal amount of dietary fat in would range about 30%; in contrast, a "high-fat" diet for a horse would constitute about 7%-10%.

Oil supplementation in the horse's diet can serve two functions: that of providing energy, in which there does not seem to be a significant difference between types of oil; and that of providing anti-inflammatory and anti-oxidant properties, which are derived from omega-3s. Again, as stated above, the horse that is kept according to ecologically sound principles will achieve very sufficient levels of omega-3s. It should also be remembered that fermentation in the horse's hindgut produces short-chain fatty acids (SCFA) which serves as a source of energy. For the older horse or one that needs additional weight gain, especially in colder months, the addition of oil to the diet is much preferable to adding more starch. For energy needed in the performance sector, dietary oils are also much preferable than added starch. Oils can deliver "cool" energy as they do not produce as much heat as do carbohydrates during digestion; high fat diets have been shown to increase both aerobic and anaerobic performance, delaying muscle fatigue. (Ahma n.d.) It should be noted that heat processed oils are virtually void of any essential fatty acids.

There is some amount of caution suggested in feeding dietary fats to horses over and above what they would normally get from a raw diet. There is some indication that glucose intolerance and insulin resistance can occur in ponies that are supplemented dietary fat exceeding their individual requirements. (National Research Council 2007) While most of the studies showing "benefits" of fat supplementation in horses have been of short duration (less than three months), Pagan et al. (1995) did a study in Thoroughbreds that lasted seven months with no adverse effects at a rate of 12% of digestible energy (DE). Another study (Harris et al. 1999) showed that 20% dietary fat supplementation caused no adverse effects after six months. (National Research Council 2007) The first two studies (the one in ponies and the one in horses by Pagan) apparently used soybean oil; the last mentioned did not designate the particular type of oil. I would caution, however, that the duration of these studies may not be long enough in the heavier breeds; metabolically it may take longer to show adverse effects in horses versus ponies. Based on this author's work, there is also some indication that soybean, being a phytoestrogen (not to mention mostly grown from genetically modified seed), may have influence in the processes that can lead to insulin resistance via its influence on endogenous estrogen; this work is ongoing and is considerably beyond the scope of this book, but is mentioned here just to make the student/reader aware of the possibility and to use caution in any dietary fat supplementation (as caution should always be used in any type of supplementation).

Linseed, palm, and soybean oils seem to be the more widely used oils in feed concentrates for adding "fat"; palm oil seems to be preferred for pelleting as it has a higher melting point. (Hallebeek and A.C. Beynen 2002) (Palm oil is one of those non-animal fats in temperate climates with a melting point of about 33-39C, according to www.Palmoil.com/ useful_info.) Of course, corn oil has been used for many years especially in the racing sector as a top dressing. Canola oil is becoming more prevalent in use in horse feeds in North America; while canola was originally developed (from the rapeseed plant) using traditional plant breeding techniques, a very significant portion of the canola now grown is from genetically engineered seed; the same can likely be said about soya and corn seed. The issue with adding oils to processed feeds is the time to rancidity, therefore vitamin E is typically added as a preservative (the use of natural or synthetic E depends upon the manufacturer); chemical preservatives may also be used. If one is top dressing the feed with added oil, then a quick "sniff test" should tell whether or not the oil is rancid.

4.5 PROTEIN

There seems to be a lot of "myth-understanding" concerning protein requirements and how they function in equine nutrition - and for that matter in the human realm as well, although that has greatly improved over the past few years, and from which research we can learn to some degree with regard to equine nutrition, keeping in mind the differences between herbivores and omnivores. Proteins are among the most complex of all organic compounds, many of them being extremely large molecules. (Alcamo and Schweitzer 2001) The term protein comes from the ancient Greek word, "protos", meaning "first". Proteins can be broadly classified as such: (Macleod 2007)

▶ Structural – the main constituents of the organism, and include collagen and keratin

▶ Enzymes – those functional proteins that catalyze cellular biochemical reactions and affecting the rate of reactions within the body; all known enzymes have a protein part; however not all proteins are enzymes; only those proteins that are capable of catalyzing a biochemical reaction are enzymes

▶ Hormones – such as insulin; they are chemical messengers affecting metabolic processes

▶ Immune compounds – are carried in the blood assisting with immunological reactions

▶ Transport compounds – assist in the transport of nutrients; hemoglobin is one that carries oxygen from the lungs to tissues

Protein is the second most abundant substance in the body after water, making up about 17-19% of the body and constituting three-fourths of the dry weight of most body cells. (Macleod 2007), (Braverman 2003) So, while protein as a dietary nutrient is not a primary source of heat and fuel (caloric energy) in the horse, being drawn upon typically only when carbohydrate and fat reserves are too low, they are involved in the growth and development of all body tissues as well as reproduction and immunity. Therefore, the amount of energy that protein contributes to cellular processes cannot be ignored and without it life would not happen.

Proteins are synthesized in various organisms (plants, animals, etc) in almost a "reverse digestion" process; i.e. through the removal of water molecules as opposed to hydrolysis in which water is added to facilitate digestion. While the intricate details of the biosynthesis process required to make protein is considerably beyond the scope of this book, in simple terms it is the genetic coding of a particular cell that provides the information on how to build a particular protein that is needed, which happens through a two-step process called transcription and translation. It is during the translation phase that various amino acids are assembled in a specific sequence to ultimately make a particular protein depending upon the function required. Interestingly, methionine is always the "start" amino acid during translation; this is found to hold true in protein synthesis in all eukaryotes and can thus be viewed as an example of the unity that exists between living organisms. (New World Encyclopedia contributors 2008UTC)

The structure of amino acids is fairly simple, having an amine group at the core and a carboxyl group with a side chain attached. It is this chemical compound side chain that determines which amino acid it is. The amine group of one amino acid and the carboxyl group of the adjacent amino acid are linked together by the removal of the molecules of water (a process known as dehydration synthesis) to make a polypeptide (a peptide bond being the strong chemical "glue" that holds the two amino acids together); one or more polypeptide chains are then combined (folded) to make a protein molecule. Small proteins are often called peptides; the word 'peptide' comes from the Greek peptos meaning 'cooked'. Many of the short-chain peptides are absorbed directly into the bloodstream. (Braverman 2003) Amino acids are composed of hydrogen, oxygen, and carbon as are carbohydrates and lipids (in differing ratios); however, amino acids

It is important to note that protein production in plants is a biosynthesis, not a direct photosynthesis process as with the production of sugars and starches. This process in plants (i.e. rangeland and pasture species with regard to horses) is directly dependent upon the vitality and health of the soil. Grazing animals are primarily dependent for their health and nutritional well-being upon the quality of organic matter that is produced as a result of the fertility of the soil. In other words, grazing animals are indirectly dependent upon a fertile soil with sufficient inorganic minerals and microbial activity in an indirect way. (Albrecht 1975) also contain nitrogen in their amine group. It is the nitrogen that allows the building and repair of tissue (Braverman 2003), but can also contribute to the "ammonia" smell in the urine soaked bedding of stabled horses when excessive protein is consumed. Many amino acids also contain atoms of sulfur (methionine and cysteine being the only two that are found in proteins) and phosphorus; some contain trace elements. (Alcamo and Schweitzer 2001) So in essence what the body is doing when dietary protein as a whole is ingested is breaking it down into the individual amino acids and then reassembling them back into whatever types of proteins are needed in the body at any given time. This is a process in which the amino acids are used up and the body therefore requires a continual supply of all amino acids, some of which are readily synthesized (assuming a healthy body), the remainder of which must be supplied in the diet (see below for essential amino acids).

Pepsin is the enzyme that begins to digest dietary protein in the horse's stomach, followed by the highest level of digestion in the small intestine via pancreatic proteases. As we saw in a previous section, proteins that pass to the hindgut are largely utilized by the fermentative microbes themselves and are generally not available to the horse. To date there are 22 amino acids; 21 of them are found in eukaryotes and 20 are directly encoded by the universal genetic code found in all but a few organisms (Wikimedia Foundation Inc 2012) – these 20 being what many refer to as the "standard" amino acids. So the animal's requirement is actually for amino acids, not "protein" per se. With the exception of lysine, there are no established amino acid requirements in the horse; however there are 10 that are presumed to be essential based upon the horse being a non-ruminant (other amino acids may be synthesized in the horse): arginine, histidine, isoleucine, leucine, lysine, methionine, phenylalanine, threonine, tryptophan, and valine. (National Research Council 2007) Some non-essential amino acids can be synthesized in the horse's body from the essential ones, a process known as transamination. (Macleod 2007) It should be noted that even so-called non-essential amino acids can become essential during periods of stress - including disease states, exposure to environmental pollution, age, as well as the use of drugs (Braverman 2003). A limiting amino acid is defined as one that is present in less than adequate amounts which may result in limitation of the synthesis of a particular protein. As well, all the amino acids required for a particular protein must be present at the same time or building of that particular protein will stop completely. (National Research Council 2007) The limiting amino acids in horses seem to be, in order: lysine, methionine, and threonine; some references will list threonine as the second of only two limiting amino acids. The fact that cereal grains, which are commonly fed to horses, are typically low in lysine likely has some bearing on that amino acid being the first limiting one. Obviously, more work needs to be done in this area; there seems to be as many if not more questions than answers.

When we speak of the quality of dietary protein, we are speaking of the amino acid composition (i.e. profile) and the digestibility of the source. Those proteins that supply all the essential amino acids are known as complete proteins. Supposedly most of the complete proteins are ones that horses typically do not eat such as foods of animal origin (meat, fish, eggs, etc). (Macleod 2007) This seems to be a persistent myth that started with Frances Moore Lappe's original statement in the first version of her book, *Diet for a Small Planet*, in which she cautioned vegetarians and particularly vegans to combine certain foods such as beans and rice in order to receive 'complete protein' since they were not eating meat or other animal protein. Ms. Lappe herself reversed this statement in the 1981 edition of the same book, saying that her original statement was in error, and this has since been corroborated by several other nutritionists and medical doctors. However, her original statement continues to be repeated as having scientific basis. It bears remembering that large herbivores such as elephants, once they are weaned (which the product of lactation - the milk - is indeed a source of animal derived protein), survive quite nicely on plant based proteins and have done so for quite a long time; as did horses prior to domestication. But we should also bear in mind that herbivores in their native habitats are provided a wide variety of feed choices; e.g. elephants will also eat the bark of certain trees to obtain dietary nutrients, including protein. What of our domestic horses on pasture? Most plants as well as microorganisms [such as bacteria, yeast, and molds] can make all of the amino acids. (Stewart 2001) It is this author's opinion that a sustainably maintained and widely varied pasture, not a monoculture, should provide a complete protein profile sufficient for all classes of horses.

Protein deficiency can result in weight loss in the mature horse, fetal loss in pregnant mares, and a decrease in milk production in lactating mares. Developmental pathologies have been seen in foals nursing mares that are deficient in protein. A lack of muscle mass can result from deficient amounts of protein in both the performance horse as well as the horse at maintenance. (National Research Council 2007)

According to the NRC in *Nutrient Requirements of Horses 6th Ed.*, ..."excess protein is degraded and results in an increase in urea, which will be excreted in the urine". (National Research Council 2007). It is actually the nitrogen in the protein that is excreted and which causes the "ammonia" smell common in stabled horses; it is normally an early step in amino acid degradation being accomplished by the urea cycle in the liver. This leaves behind the carbon skeleton. (Palmer 2008) This carbon skeleton is different for each amino acid and thus each will have its specific metabolic pathway of degradation. (Palmer 2008) Amino acids can be classed into two broad groups - glucogenic and ketogenic. The ones that go through the Krebs (or the citric acid - TCA) cycle are those that are glucogenic; they contribute to the non-carbohydrate synthesis of glucose, a process known as gluconeogenesis; these are most amino acids. (Palmer 2008) The ketogenic amino acids do not synthesize glucose; in humans the only two are lysine and leucine. Some amino acids are both glucogenic and ketogenic. As indicated above, gluconeogenesis typically happens when a situation of "starvation" sets in (when CHO and fat reserves are too low). But what happens when protein is fed in considerable excess of metabolic needs? This subject is apparently one of debate and ongoing research (in humans particularly). Excess protein can have a dehydrating effect on the horse; it can also affect the normal pH balance. (National Research Council 2007) There have been increased calcium loses with excess protein intakes reported in other species. (National Research Council 2007) In the exercised horse, increased levels of blood ammonia due to excess protein intake can result in a number of issues including nerve irritability and abnormal CHO metabolism. (Pagan 1998b) Protein stimulates insulin release, but it also stimulates glucagon release which has the opposite effect of insulin and thus brings glucose back into the blood. The theory seems to be that if consuming proteins without carbohydrates (as in humans eating meat based proteins only), then the insulin doesn't "know" whether to facilitate glucose or amino acid transport into cells. The horse that is fed according to physiological needs will be consuming both CHOs and proteins at the same time. This applies to "normal" consumption.

There has been some research into high protein diets for humans as a method of weight loss via thermogenesis and satiety; granted, the protein degradation process is an energy consuming one. However, I do not think we know all of the ramifications of feeding excess protein to horses, and considering the pathway to gluconeogenesis (conversion to glucose and stored as fat), I would hesitate to recommend an excessive amount of dietary protein for any horse and especially those that have already exhibited tendencies toward metabolic dysfunction. Compound that with the fact that most "extra" non-forage dietary protein for horses is derived from soy - a phytoestrogen and which is mostly a genetically modified crop now - you may have a recipe for disaster sooner or later. That being said, it has been my experience there is some amount of "wiggle" room in the crude protein percentage recommendations, depending upon the individual's needs and the ecology, and providing the source of protein is a clean, non-GMO one.

There are some undying "myths" concerning protein, not the least of which is that too much protein can cause laminitis. Most sources now say that carbohydrates are the culprit and not proteins. The problem I find with totally dismissing any protein/laminitis link is the source of the protein and the amount, as just discussed.

Obviously the bottom line here is to make sure the horse is getting a sufficient amount of protein given the particular needs but not in excess of those needs to the point of imbalance. Most of the information provided to horse owners has typically approached protein as a total minimum percent of feed or preserved forage (hay). This 'crude protein' (CP) measurement is a function of how much nitrogen is in the feed.[7] Such as for concentrates, one can typically find 10%, 12%, 14%-18% feeds in the form of a pelleted ration or sweet feed. Given this approach, this is a typical protein value requirement of horses:

- ▶ Mature horses/most classes -   10%-12%
- ▶ Brood mares & yearlings -   14%-16%
- ▶ Foals/weanlings -   16%-18%
- ▶ Seniors -   apprx 14%

While this is a quick and understandable approach for horse owners, it does not really address the horse's true need for essential amino acids. Additionally, too much emphasis has been given to just the protein content of a given feed, disregarding many of the other necessary nutrients. Nitrogen can come from many sources, including those which may be less than desirable, and which the source is generally not readily determined from a feed label. A few sources are beginning to recognize the flaws in the established CP designation of horse feeds, but until much more is determined as to the individual amino acid requirements in the horse, the existing measuring protocols will likely persist. I do not think that anyone is suggesting at this point that the percentage based crude protein measurement be completely disregarded. An ideal protein – a concept that considers both correct amounts as well as ratios - is a concept that has been developed and is in use in swine and poultry nutrition, but has yet to be developed for horses. There is an assumption that the ideal protein would closely resemble the amino acid profile of muscle tissue in the animal. (National Research Council 2007)[8]

---

[7]   Non-protein nitrogen (NPN) sources can also be used to bolster this measurement. Sources of NPN can be chemical additives (such as urea), chicken wastes, etc. NPNs are not generally found in horse feeds as hindgut fermenters do not have the capability of processing them, and are found more often in feeds for ruminants.

[8]   The 6th edition of the NRC's Nutrient Requirement of Horses now employs a daily feeding rate based upon body weight, energy requirements, and lifestyle, so as to create more individualized feeding recommendations. There is a free web-based program for those who may be interested in using: http://nrc88.nas.edu/nrh/

Based on a percentage measurement, pasture typically contains all the protein that any class of mature horse will need (with reference to the above requirements); and as was previously discussed, the amino acid profile is typically complete. This assumes a varied pasture of many different herbages (preferably native) and not a monoculture. Depending upon what species are present, the time of year, and the weather, CP levels of some pastures can reach as much as 18-20% on a dry matter (DM) basis.[9] What is being fed in addition to pasture, if anything, is also of great importance with regard to total protein and must be considered in the overall feed program. The following is a brief discussion of some sources of protein other than intact pasture.

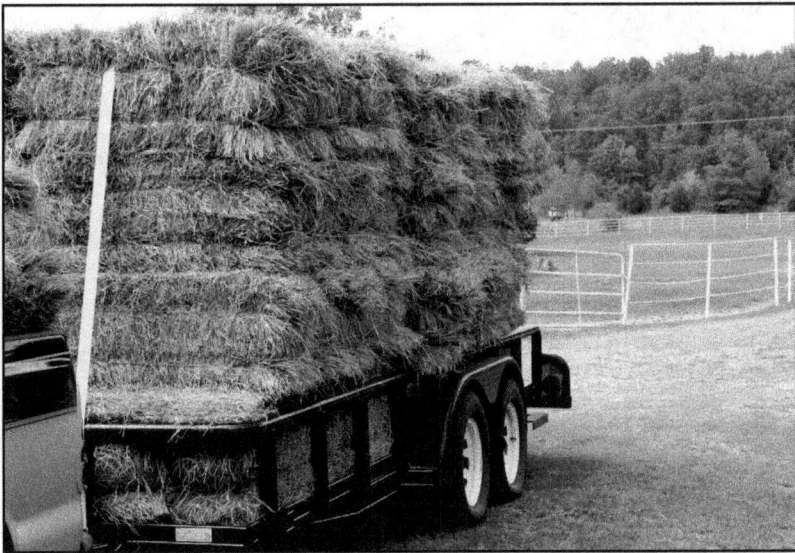

Figure 13: Load of Bermuda hay
Shutterstock image # 2136352 © Karen Givens

---

[9] A measurement of dry matter basis is used to facilitate comparison of nutrients between feeds. The nutrients are contained within the dry matter and so the physical quantity of nutrients will not change with the addition of water. However, the addition of water does change the percentage of nutrient in the overall amount of food being fed, and so the percentage of a particular nutrient in the feed will decrease with the addition of water. In other words, if it were possible to feed everything on a DM basis, you would be feeding considerably less in quantity of everything. Most forages and certainly pastures have varying amounts of water content; dry grass hay will typically contain ~10% moisture; haylage ~ 55%; silage 60-70%; and pastures, of course, will vary with the season and local weather. So if you are feeding a haylage - such as alfalfa - that contains 20% protein on a DM basis, you would certainly need to look at the "as fed" protein basis before going into a panic that you are feeding excess protein; the likely scenario of an "as fed" protein content of an alfalfa haylage is generally about 9% due to the high water content. This is an excellent website for understanding this information: http://www.ianrpubs.unl.edu/epublic/pages/publicationD.jsp?publicationId=1398.

Grass hay (dry) - the CP of grass hay is dependent upon the stage at which it is harvested. Below is a table of USDA quality guidelines for grass hay. Also refer to the short discussion on hay in fn6. It is obvious that the earlier the hay is harvested, the higher the CP%. CP content can temporarily increase in some types of hay within a couple months of storage due to decrease of the total NSC (may be dependent upon storage conditions); this is a temporary situation and CP is expected to decrease approximately 0.25%/month during storage due to volatilization. The interior of the bale will retain more protein and overall nutrients than the exposed outer surface. (Lemus 2009) Some of the more typical types of grass hay fed to horses include Bermuda, Coastal, Timothy (sometimes grown with Alfalfa and harvested in a mix), Orchardgrass, and Tall Fescue.

Quality Grade	Crude Protein %	Physical Description
Supreme	[not given; in practical terms when buying grass hay, premium and supreme mean about the same thing]	Very early maturity, pre-bloom, soft fine stem, extra leafy; indicative of high nutrient content; excellent color, free of damage
Premium	>13	Early maturity, pre-heading, extra leafy, fine stem; indicative of very high nutrient content; green and free of damage
Good	9-13	Early to average maturity, early head, leafy, fine to medium stem; free of damage other than slight discoloration
Fair	5-9	Late maturity, head, moderate or below leaf content; generally coarse in stem; may show light damage
Low/Utility	<5	Very late maturity, mature head, coarse stem; includes hay with excessive damage and heavy weed content and/or mold; defects identified in market reports when using this grade of hay

Figure 14 Table of grass hay grades
Source: http://extension.oregonstate.edu/catalog/html/sr/sr1056-e/4table1.pdf

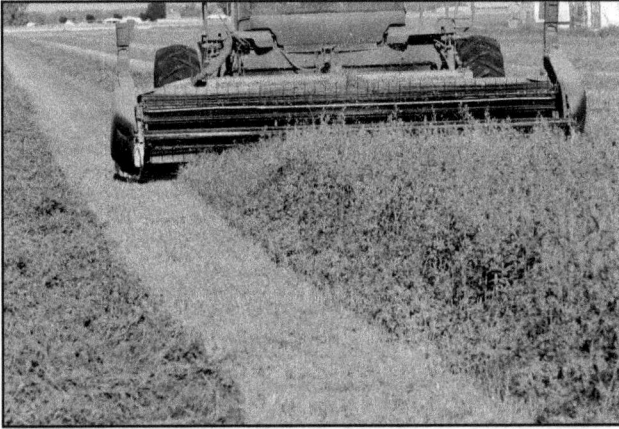

Figure 15: Mowing alfalfa
Source: Shutterstock.com image # 59528317 © Richard Thornton

Legume hay (dry) - the CP of legume hay is also dependent upon the stage at which it is harvested. Below is a table of USDA quality guidelines for alfalfa hay. The most common legume hays fed to horses include alfalfa and clover; some people will mix legume hay with grass hay for various reasons, not the least of which is to cut down on the amount of protein. There seems to be either a "love it" or "hate it" relationship with alfalfa hay among horse owners. You may hear alfalfa referred to as being "too rich"; for many people - this typically means too high in protein. Dry alfalfa hay, as indicated in the table below, can indeed be quite high in protein depending upon the stage at which it is cut. Alfalfa is a deep growing legume and thus is capable of pulling up a considerable amount of nutrients (minerals), assuming the soil it is being grown in is not depleted. This can make alfalfa extremely nourishing hay. With regard to the protein content of dry alfalfa, my personal recommendation is that feeding it in moderation with grass hay (perhaps 25:75 ratio alfalfa to grass) is a very safe approach, which can certainly be adjusted as needed.

Quality Grade	Crude Protein %	Physical Description
Supreme	>22	Very early maturity, pre-bloom, soft fine stem, extra leafy; indicative of high nutrient content; excellent color and free of damage
Premium	20-22	Early maturity, pre-bloom, extra leafy, fine stem; indicative of very high nutrient content; green and free of damage
Good	18-20	Early to average maturity, early to mid-bloom, leafy, fine to medium stem; free of damage other than slight discoloration
Fair	16-18	Late maturity, mid to late-bloom, moderate or below leaf content; generally coarse in stem; may show light damage
Low/Utility	<16	Very late maturity, mature seed pods, coarse stem; includes hay with excessive damage and heavy weed content and/or mold; defects identified in market reports when using this grade of hay

Figure 16: Table of legume hay grades
SOURCE: http://extension.oregonstate.edu/catalog/html/sr/sr1056-e/5tables.pdf

Haylage/Silage - can be either grass or legume, or a mixture of both. While both contain considerably more water than regular dry hay, silage usually contains the most with a moisture content of 60-70%. Haylage typically has a moisture content of about 55%. While some individuals may make their own haylage or silage, there are only two companies in North America that I am aware of that make haylage on a commercial basis. One is Chaffhaye, based in Dell City, TX, and the other is Tri-Forage Horsehae located in Ontario, Canada; both make haylage as silage typically contains too much moisture to be able to obtain a good fermentation without the issues of mold in a packaged product. Haylage has been used rather extensively in the UK and surrounding areas since the 1970's when Mark Westaway developed a product called Horsehage. Due to the way haylage is produced and "put up" (i.e., bagged), the guidelines in the above two charts are mostly irrelevant; all of the hay from these two companies at least is of premium quality. Please see fn9 for a brief discussion concerning the protein content of haylage, especially of alfalfa haylage.

Concentrates/processed feeds - soy is probably the most common source of protein incorporated into concentrate feeds in todays' market. It has a typical overall protein of 44-48% and appears to be valued as well for its lysine content. Canola is another meal used, having a nutritional profile close to that of soy; its protein is about 35-44%. Linseed meal is another by-product (of flaxseed) used in concentrates for protein, with levels of about 33-35%. Linseed contains significantly less lysine than soy or canola. (source: http://www.horsefeedblog.com/2011/11/protein-ingredients-in-horse-feed/). The high protein levels will be decreased on an as fed basis with consideration of the other ingredients as well as recommended feeding ratios. It should be remembered however, as mentioned previously, almost all of the soy and canola crops grown in the United States are from genetically engineered seed.

Even though horses in a non-domestic situation (i.e. open range or feral horses) are capable of moving a considerable amount in any given 24 hour period that movement is generally steady requiring low energy, with relatively short bursts of speed in situations of play or fleeing a perceived danger. The modern domestic equine athlete has high energy demands placed upon him, far exceeding those of his distant ancestors or his non-domestic range cousins. Even though protein is not a primary fuel source for energy, it is important in rebuilding the tissue breakdown that occurs during any type of exercise; it would appear that this tissue-regeneration capability would be more urgent in horses under greater sustained physical demands than what the feral horse experiences. Therefore, so long as the equine industry continues to place the emphasis upon the performance sector, the source of protein for the horse is of greater importance than what it might be for their non-domestic cousins, and thus the continued practice of feeding concentrates. Likely due to the devastating metabolic issues that can be associated with force feeding grains (for increased protein sources), there at last are some studies being done to evaluate forage-only diets for performance type horses. One study (Source: http://ker.equinews.com/article/forage-only-diet-evaluated-exercising-horses) at least showed some promising results. (Kentucky Equine Research Staff 2012) It is interesting to note that the study referred to in this article used haylage as the forage for the experimental group. Commercial haylage has the potential to be an extremely nutrient dense product that can deliver a good source of energy for even performance horses (within reason) - if it is grown and harvested properly.

For the sake of additional protein alone, one might want to consider other alternatives such as supplementation with blue-green algae, pumpkin seeds, chia seeds, or bee pollen, all of which are complete proteins (bee pollen actually contains all 22 amino acids) and most horses enjoy them; free choice clean kelp meal is also a good supplement, although it may be a "limited" protein.

4.6 SALT, MINERALS, AND VITAMINS

When we talk about minerals for livestock, including horses, many people automatically think of the mineral or salt block. One can buy a salt-only block (white); one with various minerals added (usually brown to red in color); a sulphurized block (primarily salt with only sulphur added - typically yellowish in color); or a "sweetlix" block with various vitamins and minerals as well as cane molasses and typically soybean hulls and/or some other type of binder and generally for use in cattle. These types of blocks are not suitable for horses if only because they have smooth tongues and may run the risk of either giving up and not getting enough salt or of causing some dental (TMJ) issues from trying to chew their way through the block.

4.6.1 SALT

Let's address the topic of salt only first; salt is as important to the body as is water. Sodium regulates electrical charges throughout the body and levels that are too high or too low will cause abnormalities in those signals. (Brownstein 2006) Refined salt is what the salt industry refers to as evaporated salt. Refined salt and even some sea salt are mechanically harvested. The commercial salt industry is after sodium chloride only; the minerals that are inherent in natural salt deposits are viewed as "impurities...

not necessarily detrimental to the salt's intended use, but not contributing to the benefit of salt". (Source: http://www.saltinstitute.org/Production-industry/Production-technologies/Evaporated-salt-refined-salt) Thus they are removed, typically by use of chemical treatments that may include sulfuric acid or chlorine. (Brownstein 2006) The water is evaporated under high compression and heat, disrupting the molecular structure of the native salt; then most of the water is removed. (Brownstein 2006) "When it rains, it pours"...up to 2% of food-grade refined salt can contain anti-caking, free flowing, or conditioning agents, which may include sodium ferrocyanide, ammonium citrate, and aluminum silicate. (Brownstein 2006) The free-flowing agents may not be particularly harmful in the overall scheme of nutrition, but they certainly do not confer any benefits. In iodized salt, dextrose (refined sugar) is used as a stabilizer to keep the iodide in the salt. (Brownstein 2006) The iodide in typical refined salt for human use is ~.01%. These ingredients are mentioned as some people, understanding the issues that formed blocks of salt can cause horses, will simply use loose common table salt. This author has heard more than once the comment from horse owners' as well as equine professionals that the horse's only requirement for salt is with reference to sodium chloride, nothing more; the concept of bioavailability and what happens energetically when the molecular structure is changed appears to be not be understood, or is thought to not be a viable factor in nutrition. The reasons for refining salt are the same as the reasons behind much food processing - long shelf life (i.e. no living organisms in the food to go bad); white salt is cleaner looking and thus has greater marketability; and the belief that the refining process will remove any toxins allowing mining in polluted areas. Chemically pure sodium chloride did not exist prior to the industrial revolution; it is in no way "natural" and is a man-made product. Refined salt can exacerbate mineral deficiencies within the body, and mineral deficiencies will increase the severity of chronic disorders. (Brownstein 2006)

Unrefined salt, on the other hand does not have the added chemicals, nor is it "pretty" like white table salt, but it does have all the minerals and elements associated with its place of origin. It is essentially a whole food, and there is a long history of natural salt being highly valued. Unrefined salt is either greyish in color (Celtic salt); pink (Himalayan salt), or reddish (Redmond salt). Celtic salt is "farmed" off the coast of northwest France basically as it was by the ancient Celts over 2000 years ago. These are some of the most pristine waters remaining in the world; additionally, the salt water is filtered through natural marine wetlands. True Himalayan salt comes from mines within the foothills of Pakistan. Redmond salt comes from ancient salt deposits near Redmond, Utah. The horse owner should be aware that so-called "sea salt", if it is not authentic "Celtic salt", is most times nothing more than table salt in "rock" or fine form, having been through the same refining process as the famous "pours when it rains" salt.

If there is a deprivation of salt, the kidneys will work extra hard to hold onto salt in the body resulting in eventual kidney problems; further deprivation can lead to toxic cells. (Brownstein 2006) On the other hand, it is often said that horses can eat too much salt if allowed access free choice, and that it should be fed in regulated amounts. It is my own policy to never force feed salt except in very specific therapeutic situations and then only using an unrefined salt such as Celtic or Himalayan (which, thankfully, I've not as yet had a need to do). It is my opinion based upon an ethological understanding as well as direct experience that horses in a stressed environment (and that basically means any non-native environment) can indeed eat more salt - refined or unrefined - than they need if allowed access free choice; this is a behavioural response to the environment and, again in my opinion, can stem from either a learned response (such as that from boredom), or a behavioural one resulting from a biophysical need, or both. The caveat is that most concentrated feeds contain some amount of salt to enhance taste and this salt is of the refined type. Will horses ingest more salt than they need if fed concentrates *and* given free access to salt - of any kind? My educated "guess" is that this could happen although I have not personally tried it. Feeding concentrates (processed feeds) in periodic meals is completely foreign to the horse's physiological instincts, they have no innate "reference point" with which to balance and this behavior has potential to carry over into all other dietary aspects.

4.6.2 MINERALS

This section on minerals probably took as much time to research as did half this entire book! While it may be easy enough to come up with data on the known mineral requirements of horses (and there are several as yet unknown), coming up with valid data on what *form* those minerals should be in when supplemented nutritionally was a true adventure. There is far too much marketing hype concerning mineral supplements and not nearly enough valid data; perhaps because minerals have only fairly recently begun to become recognized as vital nutritional components by mainstream nutrition. The primary forms in which mineral supplements are marketed include colloids, amino acid chelates, and ionic minerals. There is another form, called tissue or biochemic cell salts, which we will also look at. In order get a better understanding of these various forms, perhaps a basic understanding of minerals in their raw, natural form will help.

All minerals are made up of Earth's elements. Elements are the building blocks of all matter; they consist of only one kind of atom and cannot be chemically decomposed. Most minerals are compounds of elements while some minerals are single elements, such as gold and copper. Minerals are not "rocks", but they form rocks. In summary, a mineral must possess the following characteristics to be defined (as per current standards) as a mineral:

1) be naturally occurring

2) have a crystalline structure

3) be of inorganic origin (more on this aspect below)

4) possess a chemical composition

This is a brief outline of mineral classes:

(Source: http://www.rocksandminerals4u.com/mineral_classification.html)

▶   Silicates - the largest class of minerals; silicon is the most abundant element of the Earth's crust next to oxygen; they are metals combined with silicon and oxygen; mica is one example

▶ Non-silicates - the second largest grouping of minerals; these are further sub-divided into the following:

- ▼ *Native elements* - those consisting of a single element such as sulfur, carbon, gold, copper, silver
- ▼ *Oxides* - based upon divalent oxygen (metal combined with oxygen); the most common is hematite (the "rust" found on weathered rocks)
- ▼ *Sulfides* - compounds of sulfur usually with a metal
- ▼ *Sulfates* - compounds of sulfur combined with metals and oxygen
- ▼ *Halides* - small group, formed from halogen elements such as chlorine, bromine, iodine, and fluorine, combined with metallic elements
- ▼ *Carbonates* - minerals consisting of carbon, oxygen, and a metallic element; found in seashells, limestone, etc; calcium carbonate is one that is well-known
- ▼ *Phosphates* - not as common as other mineral classes; are formed when other minerals are broken down by weathering; are often brightly colored
- ▼ *Mineraloids* - substances that do not fit neatly into any of the other classes; examples are opal, jet, amber, and mother of pearl

Even though they are a relatively small percentage of the total nutritional intake, minerals are now being recognized to play a critical role in the horse's health. They perform vital physiological roles such as the formation of structural components, enzymatic co-factors, acid-base balance, energy transfer, and so on; some minerals are integral parts of amino acids, hormones, and vitamins. (National Research Council 2007) Dietary minerals are generally classified into two major groups - the macro minerals and the micro (a.k.a. trace) minerals. The macro minerals are obviously required in greater quantity (typically measured in grams per day, or kilogram in metric) and the micro minerals in very minute, trace amounts (typically measured in milligrams per day, still kilogram in metric). Going into much detail about the clinical signs of excess or deficiency in the various minerals is beyond the scope of a basic nutrition course, but suffice it to say that mineral imbalance can have far reaching impacts on health. Even trying to determine *if* there is a mineral deficiency can be a frustrating experience for the horse owner (one which I have experienced myself even just recently). Blood testing is the primary way that most equine testing is done, although hair mineral analysis has been done in the equine industry for quite a number of years (albeit many times by companies also selling mineral supplements). The issue with blood testing is that the physiology of the organism tightly regulates blood levels of minerals even in the face of pathology. High levels of toxic metals are generally only found in the blood shortly after exposure; they are moved into the tissues as quickly as possible so as to protect the blood. Blood work is a snapshot in time; as we will see below, if a mineral is supplemented in a form that is not bioavailable, it could just be "hanging around" in the blood waiting to be excreted and never make it to the target tissue, so the horse could actually have a deficiency and blood work would not reflect it. Hair mineral analysis does provide a picture over a longer period of time, but one needs to keep in mind that hair is a tissue as well and just because minerals are found in hair does not necessarily mean the body assimilated it properly (i.e. the mineral made it to the correct target site). A functional deficiency can occur even in situations of excess quantity of a mineral simply because it is not being utilized properly. It appears that hair mineral analysis is utilized often as a tool for "replacement therapy"; this is not the correct way to interpret the results and can lead to either not correcting the underlying issue or making it worse. Hair mineral analysis should be approached more from the standpoint of seeing it as a blueprint of the how the organism is responding to various stressors. Some equine nutritional professionals see hair mineral analysis as "generally not accurate". (Kentucky Equine Research Staff 1999) One vet cited a study in which horses were fed escalating amounts of calcium; the hair samples did not correspond to the increasing levels of blood calcium. (Kentucky Equine Research Staff 1999) It is not clear from this reference, however, as to the span of time between the blood testing and the hair mineral testing. If the hair sample was tested at the same time as the blood, then it would *not* reflect the increase as it would take longer to reflect in the tissue (hair) sample than in the blood. As indicated above, hair mineral analysis can and is used to detect presence of toxic minerals, but it is also now being used to detect levels of pharmaceutical drugs in the horse, with research showing that measurable levels can remain present for up to two years following systemic administration. (Kentucky Equine Research Staff 1999)

While there are basic nutritional requirements of the various minerals for horses as a species, the age and use of the animal can bear weight on mineral requirements. Generally speaking, young growing animals and broodmares require more calcium and phosphorus than the adult horse at maintenance; sodium requirements can be increased significantly during sweat loss from strenuous exercise; and so on. (Kahn 2010) Having a basic understanding of the action of the particular mineral as well as the interaction with other minerals will help the student and horse owner to understand when adjustments should be made to mineral availability. For instance, the horse that is consuming primarily a fiber diet with little to no grain *may have* a need for additional supplementation of phosphorus. Likewise, the horse eating primarily a grain diet *may have* a supplementation need for calcium. (Kahn 2010) [emphasis mine in both instances] Too much of one mineral can displace another mineral that is vying for entry to the same site. This is a list of only some mineral interactions: (Harvey 1987)

High levels of this	*Will depress levels of these*
Calcium	Manganese, Magnesium, Phosphorus, Zinc
Sodium	Potassium
Zinc	Iron, Copper, Phosphorus, Cadmium
Cobalt	Iron
Cadmium	Copper
Phosphorus	Zinc, Iron, Calcium, Magnesium
Potassium	Sodium, Iron, Manganese
Magnesium	Phosphorus, Calcium
Manganese	Iron, Phosphorus, Potassium, Magnesium
Copper	Iron, Zinc, Phosphorus
Iron	Potassium, Phosphorus, Copper

Figure 17: Table of mineral interactions
Source: Harvey, S.N., 1987. Minerals: Right on Target: Nature's Field

If the horse retains more mineral than he is losing, he is considered to be in a positive mineral balance; this is expected in the immature, growing animal as there will be accretion of minerals in various tissues. (National Research Council 2007) The mature, homeostatic horse should be in a near zero to slightly positive balance, with the slight positivity normally due to ongoing growth of tissues (hair, hooves, etc). (National Research Council 2007) Determining the state of mineral balance (+/0/-) seems to require a comparison of the amount of mineral consumed to the amount of mineral lost in both feces and urine. Collecting total output in a 24 hour period is labor intensive; therefore fractional electrolyte excretion (FE) testing is used, requiring a single urine specimen. Cross comparison between the FE test and total volumetric urinary testing, however, reveals discrepancies. (National Research Council 2007) Yet, this still does not assure that the mineral was absorbed in the targeted tissue.

Designing testing procedures to determine nutritional requirements of minerals is not straightforward with compilations of older studies used as well as extrapolations from various data; there are a number of sources for potential error. Furthermore, the calculation to arrive at the RDA for the various three major minerals required by horses - Calcium, Phosphorus, and Magnesium - used various absorption rates: 50%, 30%-35%, and 40%-70%, respectively. (National Research Council 2007) The validity of especially the 50% calcium absorption estimation is called into question: the duration of the studies (mostly less than 10 days) do not consider the high probability that the horse can adapt to lower calcium intake over prolonged periods without decrease in metabolic function. (Hintz 2001) At this point, mineral requirements for horses are primarily based upon the mature horse without any exertional influences (fetal and developmental growth, exercise, pregnancy); more research needs to be done to come to any strong conclusions for mineral recommendations outside of this. (National Research Council 2007)

As we will see below, the form that the mineral is in can highly affect absorption rates. Most NRC data seems to have been performed on supplemental, non-food sources.

The following is a brief description of the various macro and micro minerals important in equine nutrition. (National Research Council 2007) and (Harvey 1987) The Recommended Daily Allowances (RDA) are taken from *The Truth About Feeding Your Horse*, C. Macleod; the lower recommendations being from the NRC 1989 tables and the upper range being from the updated NRC tables and are based upon a 500 kg/1100 lb mature horse in light work and eating 10 kg/22 lbs dry matter per day. (Macleod 2007) I have put "RDA not stated" by any mineral that is not listed on Macleod's table (and thus not given by the NRC).

Macro Minerals

▸ Calcium (Ca) - necessary for proper formation of bones and teeth; nervous system function, blood clotting and enzymatic reactions; **RDA 25-30g**

▸ Phosphorus (P) - also a major constituent of bone and teeth; required for fat metabolism, vitamins A & D metabolism, and normal reproduction; required for energy transfer related to ADP & ATP; phosphorus is a naturally occurring element; the phosphate that Dr. Albrecht refers to is is a compound - salts containing P and other minerals; **RDA 18g**

▸ Ca/P ratio - secondarily the Calcium/Phosphorus ratio should be balanced to no less than a 1:1 ratio; if Ca is less than P, then calcium absorption can be impaired, even if there is adequate intake of Ca according to nutrient requirements for that mineral alone; the ratio in mare's milk has been reported to range between 1.8 and 2.5:1; note that horses can seemingly adapt to moderate excesses of Ca by limiting absorption and increasing excretion, a deficit however can lead to a weakened skeletal condition if the deficiency becomes severe enough, and particularly has negative consequences in foals

▸ Magnesium (Mg) - 60% is found in the skeleton and ~30% is found in muscle (assisting in muscle contraction); it is also an important ion in the blood; it plays an important role as an activator of many enzymes; is a balancing mineral for Ca, however high uptake can impair calcium uptake; **RDA 9.4-10g**

▶ Potassium (K) - it is the major intracellular cation and is involved in acid-base balance; essential for CHO metabolism, regulates thyroid function as well as body fluids; also active in nerve transmission; **RDA 31g**

▶ Sodium (Na) - critical in maintaining normal function of the central nervous system; it is the major extracellular cation and major electrolyte involved in pH balance; **RDA 30g**

▶ Chlorine (Cl) - this typically is associated with sodium in the form of the anion chloride; it is also involved in acid-base regulation; **RDA 50g**

▶ Sulfur (S) - this element is not usually found in its raw form in dietary and biological components but is obtained via the sulfur-containing amino acids, B vitamins (thiamin and biotin), heparin, insulin, and chondroitin sulfate; **RDA unknown**

Micro Minerals

▶ Cobalt (Co) - the microflora in the horse's cecum and colon use cobalt in the synthesis of vitamin B_1; **RDA 1mg**

▶ Copper (Cu) - essential for copper dependent enzymes that are involved in the synthesis and maintenance of elastic connective tissue; helps to mobilize iron stores; preserves the integrity of the mitochondria and melanin synthesis; is active in detoxification of superoxide; **RDA 100mg**

▶ Iodine (I) - found in the thyroid gland and is necessary for synthesis of thyroid hormones (T_4 and T_3); deficiencies and excesses both can limit the production of the thyroid hormones and can result in hypothyroidism; **RDA 1-6mg**

▶ Iron (Fe) - a major constituent of blood (specifically hemoglobin, myoglobin, and cytochromes) and many enzyme systems; it plays a critical role in oxygen transport and cellular respiration; caution should be exercised with supplementing iron as it tends to be one of the most over-supplemented minerals in horse feeding regimens, and most horses will get plenty of iron without supplementation; **RDA 400-500mg**

▸ Manganese (Mn) - is essential for carbohydrate and lipid metabolism, as well as for synthesis of the chondroitin sulfate necessary in formation of cartilage (part of the bone matrix); is associated with pH utilization, iron assimilation, nitrate reduction; it is necessary for normal reproduction; **RDA 400mg**

▸ Selenium (Se) - an essential component of selenium-dependent glutathione peroxidase, an enzyme with the primary biological role of protecting the organism from oxidative damage; also plays a role in thyroid hormone metabolism; has an interrelationship with vitamin E and thus assists the immune system; **RDA 1-2mg**

▸ Zinc (Zn) - is a component of more than 100 enzymes including many of the metalloenzymes (a.k.a. metalloproteins; they are proteins that contain a metal ion cofactor); the highest concentrations occur in the choroid and iris of the eye and in the prostate gland; medium concentrations occur in skin, liver, bone, and muscle; low concentrations occur in blood, milk, lungs, and brain; **RDA 400-625mg**

▸ Chromium (Cr) - plays a role in CHO and lipid metabolism; acts as a potentiator of insulin in facilitating glucose clearance (is considered essential in humans); **RDA unknown**

▸ Fluorine (F) - known to be involved in development of bone and teeth but the dietary necessity for horses has not been established (according to the NRC); **RDA not stated**

▸ Silicon (Si) - according to the *Nutrient Requirements of Horses, 6th Ed* - "Despite silicon being the second most common element of Earth's crust...surprisingly little is known about the nutritional importance of it in the diet of mammalian species." It is known to be involved in the formation of new bone and is an important component of connective tissue, hyaluronic acid, and articular cartilage; **RDA not stated**

There are other elements that in principle can be deemed essential to mammals - in extremely minute quantities as most are classified as toxic. These elements include arsenic, boron, nickel, vanadium, and so on. It should be kept in mind, however, that only in the last 40-50 years have elements such as selenium and silicon been classified as essential and have known functions (although the nutritional function of the latter still remains largely a mystery); it is my thought that every natural element has a purpose, even if we have not figured it out as yet!

Minerals are not a direct source of energy; however they are critical in their involvement in energy extraction from specific nutrients. (Ashmead 2012) Minerals primarily perform biochemical support roles. In the developmental stages, the proper balance and intake of minerals is crucial for proper formation of the body's structure - the hard tissues. This also becomes important in the re-building of these hard tissues in the adult not just in the case of physical trauma but in normal "wear and tear"; bones and teeth re-mineralize throughout life. That is not to say that minerals do not also serve important roles as co-factors of enzymes. As well, there is a significant interplay between the various minerals and other nutrients. For instance, very high levels of ascorbic acid can deplete copper but increase iron absorption due to the interaction between copper and iron (iron depresses copper and vice versa); and copper facilitates glucose metabolism. Therefore, excess vitamin C can indirectly lead to excess fat deposition in the tissues and therefore weight gain. Theoretically, we do not worry about this particular scenario with horses as they, unlike primates, make their own vitamin C… nonetheless it makes me question if a mineral imbalance would not affect the synthesis of vitamin C in non-primates.

The topic of mineral supplementation seems to vary, sometimes wildly, depending on just who you are talking to. Indeed, the entire subject of minerals in nutrition seems to be unsettled with a lot of confusing information floating around. The terms "organic" and "inorganic" have been applied to mineral supplements as a means of classification and especially determination of absorbability, and can lead to considerable confusion. Organic for many of us means "holistically grown without toxic chemicals", and with respect to "organic" food, that is true (or at least it is supposed to be!). The typical "holistic" definition of organic vs inorganic with regard to mineral supplements generally refers to the source: organic being plant-derived and inorganic being the raw state of the mineral. There are some that refer to organic/inorganic minerals with reference to those that are toxic and not, which is a bit absurd as all minerals are toxic at some level. Another definition of "inorganic minerals" is defined as all of the metallic minerals with the non-metallic ones being, well…"something". This "definition" typically lists the macro-minerals - calcium, phosphorus, etc - as non-metallic. This is also not correct as calcium is a metal yet phosphorus is not, so that definition doesn't really work either. The predominant conventional "science" view for the past 200 years or so (including the field of chemistry) has been that any substance that contains carbon is organic, and so any substance that does not contain carbon, by default, is inorganic. The issue with this approach is that there are some carbon containing minerals - diamonds and graphite for instance - that have been "historically" (according to Wikipedia) classified as inorganic ("historically" can be just as easily translated into "arbitrarily" in this situation). I personally have never viewed a diamond as an organic substance! Additionally, the minerals that are contained in plants and animals may be referred to as both organic and inorganic depending on what they are; for instance the iron in hemoglobin in mammals is referred to by some as organic, which is in direct contrast to what is defined above with reference to the metals vs non-metals. No wonder confusion abounds with regard to understanding minerals.

The bottom line is that ALL minerals are inorganic and it is not a matter of effect, quality, or origin - it is a matter of definition. (Jorgensen and Bosse 2007) Even the minerals that are embedded in plants or the body retain their inorganic properties. (Jorgensen and Bosse 2007) Just because minerals are inorganic by definition does not, however, mean they are not involved in life processes at some point, and indeed some (if not all) are vital to biological life. There is a quote by Andre Voisin in the front of Harvey Lisle's book, *The Enlivened Rock Powders*: 'The "dust" of our cells is the dust of the soil.' [Quotation marks original; quote is from Voisin's book, *Soil, Grass and Cancer*]

As we saw above, one of the ways supplemental minerals are marketed is by labeling them "ionic minerals". Many of the websites one finds when searching for "ionic minerals" give the impression that this is some major 'new discovery' that has long been suppressed, yet most of these sites do not tell you by whom or how this so-called new discovery was made. Some of the marketing hype surrounding ionic mineral supplements will include statements to the effect 'that plants absorb minerals from the soil and then convert them to this highly usable ionic form' that is being sold on the website. The problem with these kinds of statements is the most minerals are ionic by nature and no one "discovered" a new process to make them so. The minerals are in ionic form in the soil before the plant takes them up; the roots of plants absorb the minerals as ions in soil water. This is why we measure things such as cation exchange capacity of soils and perform nutrient mineral analyzes so as to determine whether a soil is properly mineralized for the health of the plant, which in turn makes for a nutritious meal for whatever animal is eating that plant. (The exception to this is a single element mineral - such as elemental copper; all elements are neutral; however they can and do form ions by transferring one or more electrons onto a non-metal. Please note that many references will refer to *all* minerals as elements, e.g. macro elements vs trace elements, which the terminology is chemically not correct but is nonetheless apparently common usage.) Ionic is the descriptive term for ion. An ion is either an atom or molecule in which electrons and protons are present in unequal numbers (i.e. they have either lost or gained electrons), giving them an electrical charge, either net positive or negative. An ion consisting of a single kind of atom is called a monatomic (i.e. can have more than one atom but must be of the same kind); an ion consisting of more than one kind of atom is called a polyatomic or molecular ion. Ionic compounds are two or more ions held together by opposite charges (i.e. electrical attraction); one being a cation (positive charge) and the other being an anion (negative charge). Cations are usually metals and anions are normally non-metals or polyatomic ions. Cations and anions "stick" together in the same way that the positive and negative ends of a magnet stick to each other. Ions can form complexes and chemical compounds quite readily and the pathway of the mineral from ingestion to assimilation can provide opportunities to interact with the immediate chemical environment. (Ashmead 2012) In other words, there is no guarantee that an ionic mineral supplement will get to where it should, and can require large doses in an attempt to make sure the mineral is being absorbed at the site it needs to be. We may hear claims that a certain brand of ionic minerals is "organic"; this probably refers to the bonding with an organic substance. According to Hans-Heinrich Jorgensen, vice-president of the Biochemical Association of Germany eV and author of *Schüssler Tissue Salts for Horses*: "There is no evidence that these combinations are metabolised any better. There is more evidence to the contrary, because these molecules are larger and the bonding with the cation even more stable. The theory that such a combination with an organic anion would penetrate a cell easier is contrary to all physiological knowledge. Absorption through intestinal membranes is regulated by the metabolic situation of the body: if there is a lack, the absorption rates increase, and vice versa decrease in case of a surplus." (Jorgensen and Bosse 2007)

Another form of supplemental mineral commercially marketed is what is called a colloidal mineral. This is what one website says about colloidal mineral supplements: "A colloidal mineral is a supplement that is capable of providing the body with certain minerals that help you maintain an optimum level of health." (Source: www.colloidsforlife.com) Another well-known website states that "organic" colloidal minerals are minerals that have been "processed through a plant and have undergone a biochemical transformation which makes them extremely absorbable (90% to 98%) and non-toxic". (Source: http://www.majesticearth-minerals.com/why.php) This is the definition of a colloid per Wikipedia: "A colloid is a substance microscopically dispersed evenly throughout another substance." For example, milk is an emulsified colloid of liquid butterfat. Put another way, it is any substance whose particle size is small enough to remain suspended in liquid or gas yet large enough to prevent or delay its passage through a semi-permeable membrane. (Milligan n.d.) In soils, nutrient minerals are "held" onto clay or humus (the soil colloids) by a static electric charge and the sites they are attracted to are negative. (Astera and Agricola 2010) When those who are selling mineral supplements tell you things like "processed through a plant", this typically means the humic shale that is in the soil. Black or carbonaceous shales contain decomposed organic matter. We should also be aware that these are the same shales that naturally contain oil and natural gas; conventional oil and natural gas comes from its migration up and out of the shale; non-conventional means employ hydraulic fracturing of the shale beds (a.k.a. "fracking") to extract the oil and natural gas that remain trapped inside the shale layers. (King n.d.) I think this begs the question of whether or not these petroleum substances have been thoroughly removed from colloidal mineral supplements. When the humic shale is mixed with water, the particle surfaces become negatively charged which allows them to bind with ionic minerals. The shale is crushed and ground to a powder like consistency then placed into large stainless steel vats; the vats are then submerged into cool water free of contaminants and kept at low temperatures for three to four weeks. The water soluble components enter the solution and the leachate or nutrient-rich layer is then siphoned off, filtered and ready for production. Depending upon the filtration process, a variable amount of insoluble particles can pass through into the final product. (Milligan n.d.) The basic concern with commercial colloidal mineral supplements is the level of both environmental toxins and toxic minerals contained in the solution, so there is a *caveat emptor* warning when buying these (indeed, all) kinds of commercial mineral supplements.

According to H. DeWayne Ashmead, "Dietary intake of a mineral micronutrient in sufficient quantities to meet dietary reference intakes does not always ensure adequate metabolizable mineral at the tissue level." (Ashmead 2012) Mineral absorption can vary widely: for instance, calcium can range from 20% to 50% of absorbability of the dose; magnesium, 25% to 75%; iron, 2% to 10%; copper, from 10% to as high as 97%; to list a few. (Ashmead 2012) This may be evidenced by an example of one particular equine mineral supplement - it contains "not less than" 3600 ppm copper while, according to the Merck Veterinary Manual, the requirement for horses is more in the range of 8-10 ppm. It is likely that high because of the form the mineral is in in the supplement (copper sulfate to be precise in this example); much more of a mineral in a difficult-to-absorb form is needed in the attempt to get some in the body. But if we understand the pathways that copper can take (as well as the influence that estrogen has upon it and vice versa), we can easily walk into a labyrinth of trying to "fix" one issue and "breaking" another. This particular mineral supplement (or similar) was supposedly formulated due to a perceived deficiency in certain regional soil levels, thus affecting the hay and pasture. However, assuming a true soil deficiency, this does not take into consideration any other aspects of the diet, of which water cannot be ignored, as well as any processed feed or concentrate being fed. The other issue we can find with such high dosing of minerals in supplemental form such as just mentioned is one similar to what we discussed with high levels of protein. And that is the excretion of much of the excess. The minerals in many equine supplements are in the form of crude mineral salts such as zinc oxide or the aforementioned copper sulfate primarily because they are lower in cost. (Kopp n.d.) These kinds of mineral salts have the least absorbability of any form of mineral; they are largely excreted adding to environmental pollution issues. (Kopp n.d.) Not to mention the fact the excreted salts are decreasing the soils nutritive value...the very soil that is trying to grow the food the horses are eating!

The concept of supplying minerals for supplementation in an ionic or covalently bound protective amino acid matrix with a stability factor that can circumvent ionization (and other absorption) issues as well as precise delivery in the intestinal brush border became a reality with chelated mineral supplements. (Ashmead 2012) They are reputedly the most bioavailable with regard to the "crude" (meaning not triturated as described below re: biochemic salts) mineral supplement forms, although one should still use caution in selecting the buying source. (Albion Human Nutrition (Ed.)) Chelates can sometimes be referred to as "organic" due to their being bound to carbon-based molecules; this does not mean they are from or produced organically (Kopp n.d.), and as we saw above, to call them "organic" is a misnomer at any rate. This protection allows the mineral to survive the acidic environment of the stomach and pass into the small intestine where it is available for absorption. The substance the mineral is bound to is called the ligand, which can be either an amino acid, peptide, or sugar molecule. The key to determining the quality (i.e. bioavailability) of chelated minerals lies with the particular the ligand used (generally should be an amino acid), including the size and making sure it is attached to the mineral in not one but two places. (Kopp n.d.), (Albion Human Nutrition (Ed.))

We talk about "bioavailability" of nutrients in nutrition. This can be defined as "…a measurement of the rate and extent of a nutrient that reaches the systemic circulation and is available at target tissue level". (Kienzle and Zorn 2006) In horses, mineral absorption strongly depends upon absorption from the gastrointestinal tract into the systemic circulation, and for most minerals this is the limiting step. (Kienzle and Zorn 2006) The particular biochemical pathways (via dietary ingestion) of mineral absorption in the horse are not completely understood as yet but absorption is believed to be accomplished through either simple diffusion, facilitated, or active transport. (Macleod 2007) Other factors can affect mineral absorption, including the chemical and structural form of the mineral, the existence of protein chaperons (enzymes are necessary for utilization of both minerals and vitamins), the individual's health status, the diet being fed, as well as any medications being utilized. (Thiel n.d.), (Loomis 2007) For instance, in a copper deficient animal iron cannot be used to build hemoglobin. (Kienzle and Zorn 2006) Mineral absorption is not the same among different species; for example, horses will excrete excess calcium in their urine while in carnivores, pigs, and ruminants, the urine is not a major excretory pathway for excess calcium. (Kienzle and Zorn 2006)

So what about these various forms of mineral supplements we've just discussed…why should we be concerned about them? Do we need to give mineral supplements to our horses? It depends, and it depends. The first question to answer really is how *should* horses (and other animals as well as humans) primarily obtain their minerals? It's simple - from food, from their natural, biologically appropriate, evolutionary diet. In a native diet, the horse would obtain most of his minerals from foraging and browsing, with some being obtained directly from the soil, rocks, etc. especially during times of drought or other times of excess need or foraging deficiency. The content and makeup of these minerals would depend upon the mineral content of the particular soil, which in turn would depend upon the geographical location as well as the micro- and macro-climate of the region; the time of year can also influence soil mineral composition and availability. This translates into...a soil that has been depleted of minerals and microbial activity through inappropriate treatment (such as use of herbicides, pesticides, too much tilling, etc) will not produce a minerally balanced "meal" (intact forage) for the horse. The renowned soil scientist, William Albrecht, said this:

> "If, in the final analysis, the soil's contribution to the plant is mainly minerals, then the more fertile soils must be fertile because they contribute more minerals. Nature has given wild animals some instincts which are demonstrated in their search and selection of feeds according to mineral supply. Calcium and phosphate as bone builders occupy first place on the animal's list of mineral dietary requirements. ... Can the legs of the horse be clean and the bones able to take the strain when built from plants which themselves are suffering lime and phosphate shortages? ... Wild animals can roam in search of their medicine, but our domestic animals, confined by fences to fields deficient in lime and phosphate, must suffer the consequences of malnutrition." [*Soil Fertility and Animal Health*, p 181]

The animal can utilize minerals in the raw form if necessary, but the plants have the ability to transform minerals into more bioavailable forms for use by animals; as well plants also provide other necessary nutrients. This is an important part of the cycle of life. The physical body is rooted in mineral consciousness. It is what makes up the biochemical aspect; it is the body's physical reality and thus any deficiencies or excesses in minerals will directly manifest as nutritional or functional imbalances. The issue we face in our current domestic equine situation (not to mention human nutrition) with regard to mineral intake is two-fold: most of the Earth's soils are largely minerally depleted as stated above; as well our management techniques for keeping the domestic horse further exacerbates ecological situations that may render mineral deficiencies. How do we resolve this? Most equine nutrition guidelines focus on forced supplementation; indeed most (if not all) processed feeds are "balanced" with various vitamins and minerals according to the current established mineral requirements for horses. Unfortunately many mineral supplements are nothing more than industrial products made from processing raw minerals with one or more acids (Thiel n.d.) resulting in mineral "salts" as we saw above. Nor does this take into account the individual - his health status, age, environment, and so on. So we can ultimately wind up with layers of feeding and supplementing regimens, each attempting to balance or correct the layer beneath.

One way we can resolve this - and this is my personal preference - is to first have your soil tested, then re-mineralize it according to what it is deficient in. This essentially means thinking "outside the box" with regard to *both* conventional farming as well as organic farming. Conventional farming basically focuses on feeding the plant that is growing in the (depleted) soil, and finding every way possible to make it more "nutritious" according to a laboratory chemical analysis (which of course ignores any aspect of life energy in the food). Michael Astera states it quite well: "The "better living through chemistry" factions are still flogging their tired horse. [*sic*] Having stripped the soil of its richness, burned out the humus and killed off the soil life, and having turned much of their not-so-little corner of Nature into a nutrient depleted toxic wasteland, they are now developing Frankenstein's monster crops, genetically modified organisms or GMOs, bred to live in these conditions." (Astera and Agricola 2010) [Quotes original] Organic agriculture tends to concentrate only on the organic fraction in soils. More organic matter is certainly fine if the soil is lacking humus, but it does not address soil nutrient deficiencies, specifically those of minerals. Biodynamic agriculture does tend to understand energy flow beyond simple electric current, and even though it utilizes some mineral preparations, it still does not completely comprehend the vital importance of minerals in the soil. The issue is that all forms of agriculture remove the plants from the soil which prevents the plants from naturally dying, decaying, and returning the minerals which the plants used for life, back to the soil. The cycle of life has been broken. The only way to remedy this is to put back into the soil the minerals which were used by the plants that were then harvested. This scenario even applies to "permanent" crops such as hay and pastureland (especially pasture that is intensely grazed) as the crop is still not allowed its decaying process. In the early stages of agriculture, farmers would allow their land "fallow" time, sometimes for years. This allowed the soil the opportunity to re-mineralize through nature's processes. While that is likely not the answer in modern times, there are ways to return to the soil the minerals that were removed by the growing plant. The complete scenario for doing this is outside the scope of this book, but suffice it to say it has successfully been done many times and in ways that are not necessarily either a financial or time burden on the farmer. In fact many farmers report decreased input costs. (Astera and Agricola 2010) Re-mineralization of pastures is a completely viable option for those who care for horses on their own property.

For those that are in boarding situations or otherwise do not have the freedom to make adjustments to their land, mineral supplementation is likely the best course. In this case, an amino-acid chelated, balanced multi-mineral (including trace minerals) supplement fed free choice is best for general maintenance purposes. When I refer to "balanced", I am referring to the various minerals being balanced among themselves; specifically balancing for the horse would require knowledge of what, if anything, the horse was deficient or excess in. There seems to be a distinct chasm among horse owners as to whether or not horses "know" when to eat free choice minerals or not. This issue is more than just cut and dried, so to speak. For those individuals that argue that horses do not have any "knowledge" of what their nutritional needs are, then I would ask the question - how do you think horses evolved over 50 million years or so to be in your barn if they do not possess any "knowledge" of what they need nutritionally (or otherwise)? For those individuals that are thoroughly convinced that horses *always* know exactly what they need and don't need - I would caution you to understand that once an animal that is part of nature is removed from his native habitat, any definition of the word "natural" is out the window. The nutritional ecology of the domestic horse can affect his behavior with regard to what we could term his innate knowledge of dietary requirements. For instance, the horse that is being fed sweet feed may very well have "lost" the ability to inherently determine his own mineral needs, if for no other reason than the biochemical mechanisms for doing so have been altered by a food that is *not* his natural diet. We find the same scenario in many mammals including humans. It is this author's experience that the domestic horse that is kept according to his ecological and ethological needs as much as possible either retains or regains this knowledge; in other words it is not lost "forever". Do I think horses should always have a good free choice mineral supplement (as described above) available? Yes. There may come times when specific forced mineral supplementation is needed, and for that I personally would rely on a specific quality amino-acid chelated mineral supplement and/or supplementation with specific biochemic cell salts. We've not talked about these biochemic cell salts yet, so let's discuss this now. However, quickly before we do so, I will mention the issue of transmutation. That is another highly debatable issue among horse owners - specifically whether or not horses - or any biological organism - have the ability to "transmute" one mineral into another. Alchemy believes it is possible; people that are not alchemists believe that it is possible; others do not. There are legitimate scientists on both "sides". At this time, my personal position is that, yes, it is possible. Can it be proven? It depends on who you want to believe. For the student that wants to read a bit more, I have provided a "discussion" on Calcium & Silicon in the concluding section.

I would only ask the reader to keep in mind that most of the attempts to prove or not prove Dr. Kervran's theories are performed in-vitro, not in-vivo (petri-dish vs living organism). The following is a brief introduction and discussion on tissue salts.

4.6.3 Dr. Schüssler's Biochemic Theory of Treatment

Cell salts, also called tissue salts or biochemic cell salts, are preparations of certain minerals based upon the science of biochemistry; they were developed by Dr. Wilhelm Heinrich Schüssler of Germany during the mid to latter part of the 19th century. While they are prepared according to homeopathic pharmaceutical principles and triturated up to a D12 potency, they are not *used* under the principles of homeopathy with regard to diagnosis and treatment as to the Law of Similars; they are used to treat deficiencies and thus fall under the Law of Opposites (contrary to popular belief, Samuel Hahnemann utilized both principles. Note that the European "D" potency is the same as the American "X" potency, both referring to decimal scale.) Any dilution past a 24X/12C exceeds Avogadro's number, so biochemic cell salts contain some amount of crude mineral substance. It should be noted that even though Schüssler referred to these minerals as salts, by giving them in a triturated form, they will: a) be completely absorbed if needed by the organism; b) if not needed by the organism they will be excreted, however the excretions will not contain any environmental toxic amounts as discussed above regarding large doses of crude mineral salts. The most common potencies that are used with animals (as well as humans) are those of D3 and D6 (or 3X and 6X); if one is concerned about "too much" crude substance, a D12 potency can be used, although I personally have never had any issues with the lower potencies with animals and prefer the lower potencies for reasons given below.

Dr. Schüssler was a homeopath as well as a general medical practitioner although he developed a preference for determining what certain mineral deficiencies (or imbalances) would cause which diseases while utilizing "homeopathic preparations" (as opposed to assessing the "totality of symptoms" picture typical of classical homeopathy). Unfortunately, his penchant for discussing diagnostic methods openly amongst homeopathic practitioners at the time did not curry favor for him. Even today, some so-called classical homeopaths eschew the use of cell salts for these very reasons, which in this author's opinion is quite a shame and a base misunderstanding of Hahnemann's principles. Always searching for a better way to help his patients, Schüssler began looking at deficiencies in the body long before the development of his biochemistry: "What is the substance that, when lacking or insufficient, will cause the disease". (Jorgensen and Bosse 2007) [Quotes original] Having been very intrigued with the work of Dr. Rudolf Virchow (known as the "father of modern pathology") Schüssler was extremely interested in attempting to determine what would trigger cells into a pathological state (he was essentially investigating cellular metabolism). Through scientific investigation, he determined that certain minerals remained in the ashes of the body after decay. Even though Dr. Schüssler became sort of an "outcast" within the homeopathic community, his training served him well; he determined that by utilizing trituration methods he could create a mineral supplement that could be utilized by the organism to a much greater degree than crude substances, bypassing the normal gastrointestinal delivery route to arrive in the bloodstream. He essentially "planted" the idea for what is now a very common pharmaceutical term - bioavailability. (Jorgensen and Bosse 2007) Even though today we have other forms of crude mineral supplementation than what was available during Schüssler's time, his biochemic minerals remain every bit as effective - and many times more so - than any mineral supplement currently on the market. It was very early in the twentieth century that Dr. Schüssler's biochemic salts were utilized by veterinary surgeons; Dr. Meinert formed what is now the Biochemical Association of Germany eV in 1902 that promotes the use of the Schüssler biochemic salts. (Jorgensen and Bosse 2007)

Remember our previous discussion of organic vs inorganic? Organic chemistry consists of the elements of nitrogen, oxygen, carbon, and hydrogen. But as we discussed, life based upon these elements alone is not possible and the so-called inorganic elements and minerals are what drive the metabolic processes inherent in organic life. Therefore, biochemistry - or the chemistry of life - describes the permanent dance between the organic and inorganic substances. It was his attempt to understand this fundamental interaction that led Dr. Schüssler to develop his biochemical cell salt theory of treating imbalances; we now refer to this interaction as cellular metabolism. It is interesting to note that the tissue salts that Schüssler determined as crucial to sustain life are the same ones that we now label as essential. (Jorgensen and Bosse 2007) His original salts consist of the cations of calcium, potassium (referred to as Kali, of which there are three: Kali mur, Kali sulph, and Kali phos), magnesium, sodium, ferrum, and silicea; and the anions of phosphate, sulphur, chloride (also referred to as muriaticum), and fluoride.

These minerals are also called electrolytes due to electrical charges that separate them. (Jorgensen and Bosse 2007) We said above that minerals retain their inorganic properties even within the organism. This does not mean they are ineffective - assuming they reach their designated sites, which as we've seen can be the issue with ingesting other forms of crude minerals. It is because of their electro-physical properties that the body is able to accomplish nerve regulation and muscle impulses, as well as fluid and energy metabolism. We can certainly understand why Schüssler referred to his biochemic salts as "functional remedies". (Jorgensen and Bosse 2007)

Schüssler's tissue salts are *not* a substitute for a species appropriate diet; the bulk of the minerals should always come from a proper diet. They should be used for general supplementation purposes when the diet is deficient in certain minerals as well as direct treatment of disorders or pathology resulting from mineral imbalance (which, of course, the former leads to the latter, however one may need to "treat" the imbalance resulting from the deficiency for a while even after the diet itself has been corrected). As we have previously seen, mineral interactions, including antagonistic effects between the various minerals, can occur quite easily. It is therefore recommended that, if more than one particular biochemic salt needs to be given, that they be dosed separately (several minutes apart should suffice given their rapid assimilation time). It is also recommended that one does not swallow the tablets whole but allow them to dissolve in the oral mucous membranes, thus delivering them directly to the blood stream. Since it is likely impossible to teach a horse to allow the tablets to dissolve under their tongue, the quantity is generally increased to offset this factor; for instance, whereas a human dose would be one to three tables, a horse's dose would be seven to ten tablets. A very effective delivery method for horses is to dissolve the tablets in water (warm water takes less time than cold) and syringe that into the horse's mouth; most horses will take to this readily, and this delivery method can require less tablets per dose. Also using a D3 potency as opposed to a D6 will deliver more actual substance in less quantity. A D3 potency will operate in the range of milligrams, while a D6 potency will operate in the range of micrograms. (Jorgensen and Bosse 2007)

Even though Dr. Schüssler originally listed his twelve biochemic salts differently, someone later put them in alphabetical order and numbered them, with the exception of Calcium sulphate, which Dr. Schüssler had eventually excluded but his followers retained. (I believe that the American listing for Calc sulph is #3 thus moving all the others down, while in Europe it remains as #12.) The biochemic salts are many times referred to simply as the number: (Jorgensen and Bosse 2007)

1) Calcium fluoride

2) Calcium phosphate

3) Ferrum phosphate

4) Potassium chloride

5) Potassium phosphate

6) Potassium sulphate

7) Magnesium phosphate

8) Sodium chloride

9) Sodium phosphate

10) Sodium sulphate

11) Silicea (also listed as Silica)

12) Calcium sulphate

There are now an additional fifteen biochemic salts developed by pupils of Dr. Schüssler that basically completes the spectrum of minerals needed by the body as far as it is currently known. They should be utilized on a case by case situation.

It is important to understand the concepts behind utilizing biochemic salts and the properties of each particular salt, and not to just give one because of a certain "disease" in a list. Determining what is wrong with the horse from a holistic diagnostic perspective will help the practitioner or owner determine the best remedy (or remedies) to give. Again, this is a basic nutrition course and we will not get in to the particulars of pathology treatment. But for those that are interested in utilizing biochemic salts with horses, this is a very good reference book: *Schüssler Tissue Salts for Horses* by Hans-Heinrich Jorgensen.

4.6.4 VITAMINS

Vitamins are organic nutrients the horse must obtain through his normal diet or through specific supplementation; most vitamins cannot be synthesize in the body in enough quantity to support biological functions (Oke and reviewed by Lawrence 2010), with the exception of vitamin C in horses. They are defined as a group of unrelated fat- and water-soluble organic compounds. (National Research Council 2007) Vitamins are required in small amounts and thus are called micronutrients; they are nonetheless essential for life and are involved in many fundamental biological processes. (Macleod 2007) Deficiency in vitamins can result in conditions of imbalance which can lead to disease conditions, as can deficiency of any nutrient. Their requirements have been calculated using different response variables including deficiency symptoms, maximizing tissue stores, and optimization of various biological functions; therefore the requirement for a particular vitamin may differ depending upon which response variable was used. (National Research Council 2007) Higher quantities of some vitamins may be needed for optimal health. (Macleod 2007) Those vitamins that can be safely fed in higher quantities than the RDA include the water soluble vitamins as well as vitamin E. (Macleod 2007) The ecology of the domestic situation in which the horse lives can affect his need for various vitamins.

Vitamins are typically classified in broad categories as either fat-soluble or water-soluble. The tables that follow reflect the Recommended Daily Allowances (RDA) and are taken from *The Truth About Feeding Your Horse*, C. Macleod; the lower recommendations being from the NRC 1989 tables and the upper range being from the updated NRC tables; they are based upon a 500 kg/1100 lb mature horse in light work and eating 10 kg/22 lbs dry matter per day and are calculated from a deficiency variable. (Macleod 2007) If it becomes necessary to supplement any vitamin over and above the diet then naturally derived, whole food vitamins are highly recommended over synthetically formulated and fractionated ones.

Fat-soluble vitamins

These include vitamins A, D, E, and K, and are absorbed from the intestinal tract and rely on adequate bile action. Fat soluble vitamins are not readily excreted in the urine as are water soluble vitamins, being absorbed in association with fat, and thus can be stored in the body's fat tissues and liver. (Oke and reviewed by Lawrence 2010), (Macleod 2007) Vitamin overdose - a condition known as hypervitaminosis - is possible, and in particular with vitamin A. (Oke and reviewed by Lawrence 2010)

Vitamin	
A	**Function** Vision; growth; bone development; reproduction; immune function **RDA** 22,000-30,000 iu **Deficiency** Weight loss; respiratory & gut dysfunction; poor fertility; anemia; poor night vision **Excess** Can be very toxic reflecting in: bone fragility; skin lesions, reduced blood clotting; internal hemorrhages **Notes** Carotenes are not toxic and found in very high amounts in green forages

Vitamin D	*Function* Regulates Ca & P balance
	RDA 3,000 mg
	Deficiency Poor appetite; reduced growth rate, skeletal abnormalities
	Excess Toxic in excess synthetic supplementation; symptoms similar to vitamin A excess
	Notes Naturally produced from sunlight on the skin which is not toxic in excesss
Vitamin E	*Function* Antioxidant; helps in immune & muscle functions
	RDA 800-2,000 mg
	Deficiency Muscle dysfunction; cardiovascular; lowered immunity
	Excess Is the least toxic of the fat soluble vitamins
	Notes Obtained from green pasture; reasonable over-supplementation in cases of breeding & illness ok
Vitamin K	*Function* Blood clotting; protein synthesis
	RDA 10 mg - no published requirement
	Deficiency Unknown
	Excess Colic & kidney failure from excessive synthetic supplementation
	Notes The hindgut bacteria supply this vitamin

Figure 18: Vitamin requirements in horses - fat soluble

Source: Macleod, C., 2007. The truth about feeding your horse. London: J.A. Allen.

Water-soluble vitamins

Most excess water soluble vitamins are absorbed into the bloodstream and are not retained by the body once they reach a certain level, the excesses being primarily excreted through the urine; the exception to this is vitamin B_{12}, which is stored primarily in the liver. (Macleod 2007) C and the B-complex vitamins comprise this category. The horse can synthesize vitamin C in the liver and a healthy horse will have no need for supplementation. (Macleod 2007)

Vitamin	
C	**Function** Antioxidant; integrity of connective tissue; iron metabolism
	RDA N/a for healthy horses; 10 g for those with respiratory conditions
	Deficiency Not known but possibly oxidative stress
	Excess Not known; is excreted but could be a tolerance level as in humans (above which causes diarrhea)
	Notes Synthesized in the body; intense stress and respiratory conditions can require supplementation
B complex vitamins	**Function** Components of enzymes; energy metabolism & nerve conduction
	RDA B1/thiamine 50 mg; B2/riboflavin 20-30 mg; Others unknown
	Deficiency Thiamine – poor appetite, fatigue, mental depression, lack of balance; Others - unknown
	Excess Supplementation should be safe as excesses (except B12) are excreted
	Notes Obtained from forage rich diet via hindgut fermentation

Figure 19: Vitamin requirements in horses – water soluble

Source: Macleod, C., 2007. The truth about feeding your horse. London: J.A. Allen.

As we can see from these tables, the healthy horse will obtain all the vitamins he needs by being allowed free choice access to pasture and sunlight. It is when the horse's complete biological requirements are not fully met do we begin to see abnormal conditions manifest.

5

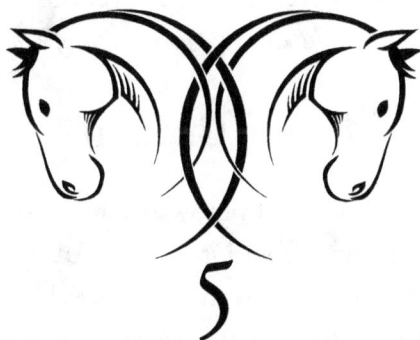

FEEDING FOR VARIOUS LIFE STAGES

ALL ANIMALS HAVE somewhat differing nutritional requirements for their various life stages, the horse being no exception.
This does not mean that the basic physiological requirements are
different; it does mean that overall quantities as well as requirements of
individual nutrient components can change in response to not just age but
external and internal stressors as well. The presence of any abnormal condition or disease can temporarily change nutrient requirements, although
it should be recognized that disease or pathological condition could very
likely be the *result* of nutrient deficiency to begin with. Addressing the
particular nutrient requirements in the face of various pathologies or other
abnormal conditions (such as orphanage) is beyond the scope of this book;
we will, however, look at differing overall nutrient requirements for various
life stages with regard to reproduction and growth - mares, stallions, and
foals; as well as the senior horse. I do not consider the performance horse
as a "life stage" but more of a classification with regard to use. We have
touched upon various nutritional aspects of performance horses throughout
this book and so will not re-address those here. It is this author's opinion
there are some deep seated ethical issues with regard to the use of horses
in the various performance sectors, the discussion of which are much too
involved and outside the scope of this book.

This is intended to be a generalized discussion; if the reader should desire a table of specific nutrient components for various classes and life stages please refer to the NRC's *Nutrient Requirement of Horses 6th Ed.*

5.1 Reproduction and Growth

"A decision regarding your foal's growth rate needs to be made early." (Adams n.d.) This is a quote from Dr. Martin Adams, equine nutritionist for Southern States Cooperative in an online article titled "*Nutrition of the Growing Horse*". (Adams n.d.) [Southern States is a distributor of several brands of processed feed including their own label.] It is indicative of an industry that is centered around and consumed by manipulating all aspects of equine nutrition for the benefit of a winning status and a marketable "product". The object is to "grow" the foal to its full genetic potential as quickly as possible to maximize income and reduce upkeep costs. Within just one particular brand on the Southern States Cooperative website, there are no less than 11 different types of equine feed listed, including pelleted and textured. There are feeds specifically formulated for every life stage of the horse, primarily based upon the percent of protein, as we discussed previously; some protein content being ~30%. Can one commercially breed viable, healthy foals without processed feed? It is this author's opinion that it certainly can be done – within the parameters of an ecologically sound breeding program. That last part is the caveat. While a particular breeding program may win accolades for producing big foals that consistently win, that does not necessarily equate to an ethically sound equine welfare program; in fact the very practice of forced breeding is diametrically opposed to sound welfare practices. In other words, adjustments are going to have to be made in order to accomplish a sound breeding program based upon the complete biological needs of the horse.

Foal nutrition begins before conception. The gestation period of a mare is approximately 11 months. Mares are polyestrus with an annual anestrus season that is triggered primarily by declining daylight hours. The majority of foals in a non-manipulated breeding environment are born in the late spring and early summer months; this allows optimum nutritional foraging for the lactating mare as well as maximum growing time for the foal before harsh weather sets in. (Goodwin 2007) This "natural" behavior is mirrored by a common (at least among Thoroughbred

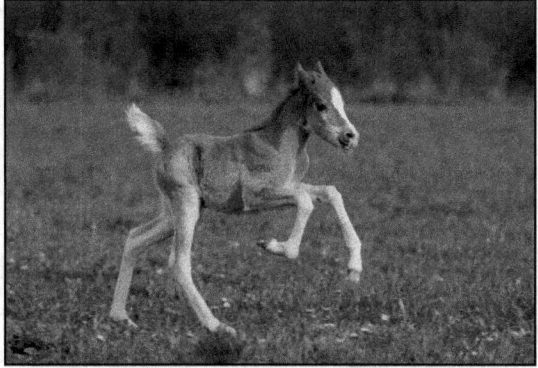

Figure 20: Young foal playing on pasture
Source: Shutterstock.com image # 100734058; © Lenkadan

farms) nutritional manipulation utilized for mares, called a 'rising plane of nutrition'. (Meunier 2012) Plane of nutrition is defined as the quantity and quality of per capita food intake, and it involves purposely maintaining the mare in a light body condition for a period of time, then bringing her condition up to more optimum levels over a period of approximately two months. This is typically done over winter into early spring. (Meunier 2012) It has the effect of triggering the mare's normal estrus cycle much as the seasonal re-growth of a native habitat would do, along with the increasing daylight hours. The issue with utilizing this technique in forced breeding programs is that processed feed is typically used (along with ignoring biologically natural mating behavior). If the mare were kept on a well-nourished pasture, this rising plane of nutrition would naturally occur in temperate climates.

The mare's nutritional requirements during the first eight months of pregnancy are not much different than of a non-pregnant mare at rest; it is during the last trimester that the fetus does the majority of growing, thus increasing the mare's nutritional needs. (Macleod 2007) Although this aspect is usually highly manipulated with supplements and various processed feeds in most breeding farms, there truly is no reason the mare cannot receive ample nutrition *if* the pasture and hay are of the highest nutritional quality and *if* there is ample pasture space for the mare to pick and choose what she needs out of a multi-species forage growth. And of course, therein lies the primary issue – the mare is typically restricted for one reason or another and/or the value of the nutritional aspect of the pasture is undervalued. The mineral nutrition is of utmost importance, so make sure the mare has access to quality free choice minerals and kelp as previously discussed. Without worrying the mare, be cognizant of her condition throughout the gestation period. Mares will typically decrease their quantity intake during the final month of pregnancy, so again, quality is of utmost importance. Lactation essentially doubles the mare's energy requirements. Relatively minor weight loss is common during early lactation periods; this is normal and the mare should not be forced into putting on more weight during this period. If the nutrition for both the mare and the foal is sufficient, she will put weight back on as the foal decreases its "pull" on her reserves.

Foals are born without their own immunity; the window of opportunity for the foal to receive the immunoglobulins from the mare is about 24 hours (Macleod 2007), which is the only time the foal will physiologically require the vitamin A rich colostrum in its lifetime (which is not to say that vitamin A is not a requirement of mature horses). If the mare is allowed to her own devices, this will typically be conferred to the foal within the first twelve hours. In non-biologically appropriate breeding circumstances, it is, unfortunately, not uncommon for the mare to reject the foal's suckling, at least initially. In these situations, the owner should be well-prepared to administer colostrum to the foal. To state that colostrum is important to the life and health of the foal is an understatement.

As stated above, the in-utero foal will have a growth "spurt" during the last trimester; this growth spurt continues for the first few weeks after birth. The foal will continue what may seem to be rapid growth, slowing down as he or she approaches maturity. (Thomas 2012) The overall long-term (genetic) growth pattern of the foal should approximate a sigmoid curve with differences among the different breeds. (Thomas 2012) The short-term growth patterns are influenced by the ecological aspects (seasons/temperature, available feed, weaning policies, the lifestyle environment, etc). The short-term growth patterns also appear to be influenced in a significant way by the time of year in which the foal was born. As was stated above, in most non-manipulated breedings the foal is born in the late spring or early summer months. Many Thoroughbred farms, for instance, will deliberately breed so that the foal is born very early in the year. Dr. Staniar of Penn State has found there is significant difference in the short term growth pattern between same-breed foals born in January vs April, with the April-born foals experiencing a greater early-on growth rate than those born in January. (Thomas 2012)

Foals will typically begin to nibble at their dam's feed (whatever it may be) at around two to three weeks of age. (Macleod 2007) For the healthy foal, there is no reason to not allow him free access to pasture with the dam. After about four months, the mare's milk becomes less nutritionally important; the foal is typically eating independently by about six months of age. If weaning is done in a biologically appropriate manner, there will be no addition or change to nutrient requirements as the weanling will adjust his own nutrition from both learned and innate behavior. Unfortunately, most breeding farms force-wean all foals, generally at around four to six months of age. Some farms will practice segregating into similar age groups so as to make it more convenient to feed; foals in this situation will typically get a concentrate specifically designed for their age group. Many foals are sold shortly after weaning. In a non-manipulated setting, mares can sometimes continue to nurse foals up to a year, with the nursing sessions becoming more and more infrequent. Starchy concentrates are just as contra-indicated for the foal/weanling as they are for any horse; the foal/weanling has the same digestive physiology as an adult horse. The primary difference between a horse that is in developmental stage and one that is mature is that the structural physiology is going through a maturation process (this is not considering any cognitive learning processes during this time, which are most certainly present; that subject is beyond the scope of this book and will be addressed in a subsequent one). It should be noted that a horse's boney structure does not fully mature until five to seven years of age depending upon breed.

With regard to stallions, if they are kept in a biologically appropriate environment, there should not be any nutritional requirements different from any non-breeding stallion or gelding. Poor sperm quality has, however, been attributed to vitamin deficiencies (Macleod 2007), so making sure that the foraging is of highest quality and supplementing when necessary is recommended for the breeding stallion. It is when we get into the typical stallion management practices that nutritional requirements can become a-typical. Unfortunately, too many stallions are kept in confinement. The stress of any biologically inappropriate environment has the capability of altering normal nutrient requirements, or at least the physiological response to what would normally be appropriate nutrition. The options are far too numerous and each situation has to be considered individually. But the obvious solution is to maintain a biologically appropriate herd consisting of the stallion and his harem with various offspring. Sadly most people do not have any idea what a "normal" equine herd looks like and stallions fall prey to a "self-fulfilling prophecy" of being labeled as aggressive and dangerous. (Skipper 2010) Far too often modern equine industry practices and the ethical and biological needs of the horse conflict, with industry practices winning out.

5.2 Feeding the Senior Horse

Senior status is variable among breeds and even individual horses within breeds, though most people consider a horse 20+/- to be senior. But that doesn't mean the horse is "old" with regard to capability. There are plenty of 30+ year olds that can run circles around the human; and in fact I have one living with me! We should go by the *signs* of aging rather than the actual age. With regard to nutritional requirements, the senior horse has no physiological differences from the younger adult. As we have previously seen, a horse 15-20 years old may begin to lose some teeth; as well, the horse that is 25+ years may begin to show issues with masticating food properly and we may see signs of "quidding". The evidence of quidding of forage will be boluses of food dropped from the horse's mouth. The longer the horse has spent his life allowed a species appropriate diet, meaning free access to forage only, the less dental issues the horse will have going into advancing age, given no other health issues. But because of the horse's hypsodont dentition, it is highly recommended that the senior horse continue to have at least an annual dental checkup and may need to be done twice yearly in some situations.

There is never any need to remove the older horse from pasture, even if he (or she)

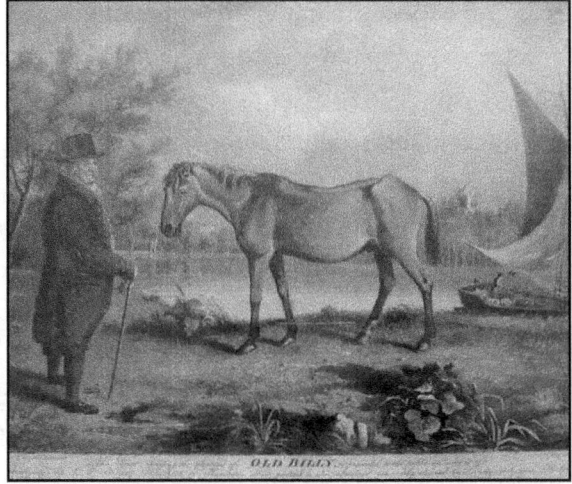

Figure 21: Old Billy, 1760-1822
Source: lithograph c.1820, author unknown

starts to quid the grass. He will still be getting some nutrients, although he will need to be supplemented; additionally the action of masticating is a biological requirement, just as it is with any horse. There will come a point that the older horse will not be able to masticate long-stem dry hay; at this time (preferably before he starts to lose condition) weaning him onto a chopped haylage product is an excellent way for the horse to obtain nutrients that he would not get otherwise. Soaked hay cubes are another excellent feed for the senior horse, although some owners are reluctant to feed soaked hay cubes because of the perceived time "cost". I personally have done so and found that if I simply put the cubes into soak while doing barn chores, the "extra" time required is virtually nil. There is no reason to not feed both soaked hay cubes and chopped haylage; the haylage can be fed free choice and the soaked hay cubes can become a "meal". In this way, between the pasture and the haylage, the horse is still allowed to trickle feed as desired and the forage "meal" should present no digestive issues; it is also an excellent opportunity to provide appropriate nutrient supplementation to assist the naturally decreasing digestive functions of the aging horse. As with any forage, the hay cubes should be of high quality. Typically one finds hay cubes in either timothy or alfalfa, or a mix of both. Which to feed will depend upon the individual horse and the availability in the local area. Some people will recommend soaked beet pulp over hay cubes. In a perfect world, I have no adversity to recommending beet pulp. However, the unavoidable fact is that most commercially grown sugar beets (the type of beet that is generally used for beet pulp; and no, beet pulp is *not* loaded with sugar) are GMO crops. Even if they are not genetically modified, the method for kill-down on the beet tops (the greens) in order to harvest the beets (the root of the plant) is to use herbicide spray. Exactly how much herbicide is going to be taken up by the root – the beet – is a variable factor that will depend upon the exact chemical compound used and its half-life. Finding organically grown beet pulp is practically impossible (if someone has a source, this author would be very interested in knowing it). This simply is not a risk I personally am willing to take. This is not to say that the hay grown for the hay cubes has not had herbicide applied to the field, although it is generally not applied as often to hay fields as it is to commercial beet crops. It may be quite possible to find a hay cube product that is at least somewhat sustainably grown, at least easier than finding organic beet pulp!

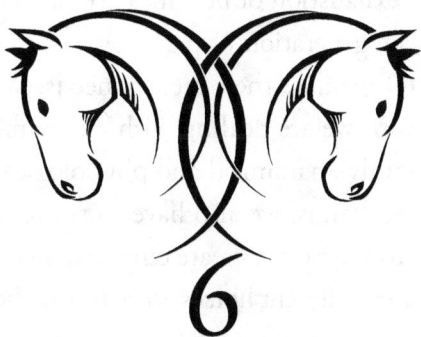

6
CONCLUSION

WHAT HAPPENS WHEN you are forced to do something that is completely different than what you are used to or have known? Do you rebel or do you simply submit? Your cognitive reaction probably depends upon what you are being forced to do. Horses definitely have cognitive abilities, but their reactive processes as well as their desires are not separate from nature as is ours. What this means when we force feed a horse in ways that are foreign to their natural physiological requirements, something suffers. And that something is either going to be their health or their behavioral response - or both. There is another "kind" of behavioral response … when we think of "behavioral" response, we tend to think of an immediate reaction to a stimulus; but it can also include the "behavior" of the physiology. We tend to think of physiological processes as "dumb" or automated processes. In other words, we assume there is no cognition involved … not cognitive in the way we think of conscious thought processes. But what if the physiology does have some kind of cognition? Some kind of *re*-cognition (i.e. recognition)? When we feed appropriate foods, the body responds by a state of health and homeostasis. When we feed inappropriate substances (which are not worthy of being called "food"), the body responds with a state of trying to cordon off and getting rid of these "invaders". If we keep throwing these inappropriate substances into the organism, after a while of fighting it either gives up from exhaustion or becomes armored, or both. Either way, you are looking at the generation of pathology. Horses that are force fed lose the ability to self-regulate their dietary needs. When we are dealing with a living organism, we are dealing with a dynamic individual being. While there are certainly anatomical and physiological similarities within the species of Equus caballus, we also have to realize that each horse and each individual environment can create circumstances that are unlike any other. Indeed, even two different horses co-habiting the same environment can react differently to the exact same feeding regimen.

Another little recognized aspect of nutritional biology of the horse is that they have evolved to be able to adapt to varying planes of nutrition. We spoke a little about this in the Reproduction and Growth section. Allowing the horse to actually lose weight over winter respects his natural biological processes. Western civilization tends to be obsessed with diet, and overeating is an all too common occurrence. This unfortunately carries over to the animals under our care; horse owners tend to panic when they see their horse losing some amount of weight over winter and will increase the quantity of feed to compensate. This is foreign to the horse whose not-so-distance ancestors were completely adapted to a decreasing plane of nutrition over winter. Those same horses also knew to increase their plane of nutrition prior to the onset of winter and would naturally gain weight during that time. Modern day horse owners will then respond to this with either increased exercise (to get that weight off!) and/or reduction in amount of food. All of this has the effect of being virtually the opposite of what the horse would naturally do left to his own devices.

It depends upon your viewpoint as to how you will attempt to "fix" the layers of imbalance that begin to creep forward from a biologically inappropriate diet: 1) if your viewpoint is more "conventional", you will do or give something to suppress the symptom, make it go away so it doesn't have to be dealt with; or 2) if you come from a more "natural" viewpoint, you will likely search the internet for a supplement that will address the symptoms your horse is showing. Neither option is addressing the underlying causal factor, but that is how the vast majority of horses today are managed. The only real, valid option is to return the horse to correct biological diet that respects the physiology of the species. The problem with doing so is that the human wants and desires get in the way...but most people call that necessity. So, I ask you - why is it necessary to continue racing a horse that is falling apart physically and mentally? Why is it necessary to continue breeding the mare that is showing signs of exhaustion simply because she is "valuable"? The equine industry - all aspects of it - has literally turned our horses into machines that we throw substances into which are derived from laboratory-designed nutritional values so that we can keep our horse "machines" going as long as possible. And both "sides" are just as guilty of this - meaning both the so-called conventional and alternative factions. We do not need to design another "holistic supplement"...we need to start feeding our horses according to *their* needs and desires! We have assigned human-centric qualities to our horses so that we can relieve ourselves of the guilt: "He loves to run...he ran his heart out", speaking of the race horse as he was being whipped yet one more time. Yes, he *literally* ran his heart out.

6.1 THE CAN'T SYNDROME

This is the part where I get "on my soapbox". I've been in the horse world long enough to have heard most of the reasons why a certain person's horse has to be fed out of a bag. If you are taking this course or reading this book in order to gain better knowledge to then help teach horse owners, good; but you will need to be tough, and as you will see below, it may not always be just the horse owner you need to work with. If you are reading this for your own personal use, then some of this may get a little personal. As I said in the Introduction, nothing carries any intent to offend. On the other hand, there are lives at stake ... lives that are dependent upon us humans to provide the best possible care for them. I, for one, do not take that task lightly and that task requires knowledge - it requires being able to *see*.

We often hear the following responses (otherwise called excuses) from many lay and professional people alike (regardless of whether they are "conventional" or "holistic") regarding why we "have" to ply our horses with "balanced" formulated feeds and all sorts of supplements: A) horses can't eat grass anymore without foundering and must be fed low starch feeds; B) all the hay is severely lacking in nutritional value; C) the performance horse can't possibly get enough "energy" from just eating forages; and D) (the lamest excuse of all) - "it's always been done that way". And these are only some of the more common ones.

Let's start with B) - we discussed this to some detail in the Minerals section with regard to re-mineralizing the soil to produce a nutrient dense forage product, intact or cut. I agree that it is not always easy to obtain quality forages, both intact (pasture/grazing area) and cut (hay), and that yes, much of the soil in this country is depleted. However, it can be done, and the more pressure that is put on commercial hay producers of any size to provide a quality product, the more they will do so. Start by educating the hay growers; if that is you, then there isn't the resistance factor to overcome. If you purchase your hay, then you have some work to do; if that grower won't cooperate, then find another one. Any area that produces hay will almost always have more than one grower. Commercial haylage is an extremely suitable option (again, the two companies I am aware of in North America are: Chaffhaye in TX and Tri-Forage in Canada). Properly grown and bagged haylage has the potential to retain virtually all of the nutrients at almost maximum capacity from when it was cut until it is fed; the shelf life of properly bagged and stored haylage is generally at least 18 months. Regular dry hay will lose nutrients just during the time it lays in the field while curing with additional losses during storage; haylage is typically in the field after being cut less than 10% of the time that regular baled hay is. Another distinct advantage to haylage is there is very little to no waste, as opposed to regular baled hay. If you've fed regular baled hay to horses, then you know they will eat what is the best out of the flakes and use the remainder for a toilet.

Get both the hay and the soil that grows the horse's pasture tested ... know what the mineral balances are. That is the only way you can sanely know whether or not to make adjustments to the mineral content of the soil. Some (if not many) large scale hay growers (including the haylage producers) will do this periodically because they understand their lively-hood depends upon a quality product. Ask questions, do not be afraid; if the grower refuses to answer, then he either doesn't understand or doesn't care and you can then know how to proceed. Even with a perfectly balanced hay and pasture, I have no problem recommending a quality, amino-acid chelated and balanced macro/trace mineral supplement *offered free choice*; and as was mentioned previously I would also make available a quality kelp meal free choice. The reason being, there are factors beyond our control (and likely knowledge at this point) that can cause a need for additional minerals or a change in what we have deemed "perfectly balanced". Between all of these factors, the minerals should be available to the horse as his body needs them.

If the horse is boarded and the stable provides all the feed including the hay, then you have an even tougher challenge. Many full service boarding stables have set routines and absolutely nothing will change the owner's mind. If this is the situation and the stable's routine does not fit a species appropriate life, then the only answer is to change stables and find one that does if keeping the horse at home is not an option. While most boarding stables generally do not adhere to an ecologically appropriate care routine for horses, that doesn't mean it can't be done. It most definitely can without any significant expense (so that doesn't need to be an excuse). This is one of the areas that will take a tremendous amount of re-education. The other major area for re-education lies with potential horse owners. One of the biggest issues is that too many people do not put a lot of forethought into what it takes to care for a horse according to the species' needs; and much of that comes from either too little available knowledge and/or getting the incorrect knowledge.

As for C) - the performance horse not being able to derive enough caloric energy from forages alone, it has been done and it is being done - with quality forages. There is finally beginning to be some amount of research and studies into the aspect of utilizing forages for the performance horse. The ones I have read so far are supportive of the fact of feeding forages in the performance sector with at least a reduction in grain if not complete removal. I would like to see studies utilizing quality haylage as the cut forage; given what I know about its nutrient density and its digestibility, I would have no issue relying solely on that with no grain whatsoever for sufficient caloric energy for very active horses. But remember that you can't drive your car at 100 mph non-stop no matter how much quality fuel you put in it; by the same token you cannot force your horse beyond his physical capabilities, sustained by supplements or otherwise. Unfortunately, again, human desires and wants tend to displace the welfare of the horse. And as we see time and again, the nutrition is not the only aspect to the overall wellbeing of any horse, and this is no less true for performance horses that are typically stalled for large parts of their lives because they are either too valuable or they will get dirty, or some other implausible reason.

With regard to D) "it's always been done that way" ... I am not sure it is even worth commenting on. We sometimes hear this comment in conjunction with another idiomatic saying "if it isn't broke, don't fix it". I certainly understand the lack of desire to change things that are working in seeming perfection; I tend to not bother with change in those circumstances myself preferring to concentrate on more important matters. But with regard to force feeding the horse an unnatural diet, this does not hold water. The results of those practices are far from perfection.

So what about A) - the "fact" that horses can't eat grass anymore - the stuff is loaded with sugar! As we've already seen, horses have a tremendous physiological capability to digest sugars - if they are allowed to ingest them as they are designed to - in small, trickle-fed amounts over every 24-hour period. We hear time and again that the grass is "not what it was 100 years ago". Yes, it is true the agriculture industry has formulated many new hybrids designed to fatten cattle up quickly that are intended for slaughter, and GMOs are, unfortunately, invading the forage market. But I think this begs the question of just how many horse owners have gone to the expense and trouble of ripping up their pastures or hay fields and re-seeding these specialty hybrids? Certainly large, wealthy equine farms and large commercial hay producers may do just that; but the ordinary horse owner typically does not. And the licensing hurdles one has to go through to grow GMOs is definitely not worth the effort for the vast majority of horse owners or even hay producers. Of course there is the ever-present threat of cross-contamination, and unfortunately alfalfa is one of the newest crops to be targeted for genetic modification. Further reading on this subject may be found in Appendix 2 of this book.

I am not down-playing the aspects of laminitis and founder in the least…I have and am dealing with it myself. Yes, insulin spikes have been implicated in founder (just ask the horses that gave their lives to show us that in a "well-designed" study recently). (Asplin *et al.* 2007) Once again, if you restrict your horse's natural grazing patterns, they most definitely can ingest more quantity than they may physiologically be able to handle at one time. The subject of laminitis and founder is a complicated and far-reaching one, but I think it is one within which we are not asking the appropriate questions, simply because we don't like the answers. I realize this is a very bold statement and one that I will catch a lot of grief over given what the majority of the so-called "data" implicates, but it is my opinion that it is the rare horse which is allowed continuous access to an *appropriate* pasture - with regard to both quantity of space allowed and quality of foraging (as well as otherwise appropriate care) - that will suffer the chronic laminitis and founder that we see far too much of nowadays. Not all "wild" horses live on sparse foraging as those in the western U.S.; consider the feral horses in places like New Zealand thriving on so-called "lush" pastures with no problems. (That "sparse" foraging of the desert is very likely to be extremely minerally rich which I also think is a key factor in laminitis & founder situations, meaning the lack of or imbalance of certain minerals.) Too many times, we are missing - or choose to ignore - the underlying etiologies that cause these conditions; and they almost always can be traced to inappropriate welfare and management of the domestic horse. We continue to try to fit a square peg into a round hole. We continue to try to "adjust" the current nutritional paradigm of the horse to avoid - or cover up - these conditions. But what do we wind up with? No real solution and subsequent problems to boot. Too much information regarding equine nutrition comes from academic and laboratory based research (the reductionist view) with not nearly enough observation of the horses themselves (the holographic view). As well, a very limiting factor is the lack of nutritional education within the veterinary teaching institutions, and what is taught is generally sponsored by one of the major feed companies. We simply do not need to keep tweaking the existing paradigm…we need to develop a new one, one that truly respects the horse's complete needs. [There is another aspect of laminitis and founder that I think is being ignored, one that is not directly nutrition related. And that is the practice of certain drugs being given to mares for one reason or another, especially during the last trimester of pregnancy and/or during nursing. There is the potential to affect the foal during the highly influential developmental stage which can have permanent effects upon certain organs and their hormonal pathways that may not manifest until adulthood. There is some research being done within the human sector attempting to track the progress of developmentally-induced, adult onset metabolic conditions with the evidence indicating it can indeed occur. Unfortunately, I do not think this will be done any time soon within the equine sector to a significant enough degree given the tremendous influence of the industry to maintain the status quo.]

Another response that is often given in relation to the typical modern feeding practices of horses is that they have "adapted" to their domestic situation and to be being fed "fake" food. That is about like saying that dogs have "evolved" to become omnivores (or even worse, vegetarians!) simply because of their association with humans. Neither instance bears any truth. Horses are indeed adaptable creatures – they have to be to have gone through what they have over the past several thousand years in their relationship with human kind. And, yes, the horse/human relationship is going through a major adaptive change. And, yes, we do need to try to find ways that can teach horses to become functionally adapted to his domestic environment. But this in no way excuses nutritional practices that are simply physiologically incorrect and we humans need to find ways to re-organize the equine environment so that is can honor the horse's biological (and ethological) needs. It does not mean that humans must suffer in the process. There is no reason the two species cannot become members of a fully functional heterospecific society.

The epistemic processes that we label "science" do not occur in a peaceful evolutionary flow; it is punctuated by "intellectually violent revolutions". (Kuhn 1970) Science is organized at any stage by a reigning paradigm or organizing idea, and all facts are interpreted in this light. It is when anomalies emerge that are too numerous to ignore or explain under the current paradigm that a scientific revolution occurs. It is typically those that stand on the outside of the current ruling paradigm that tend to bring these revolutions about. (Verspoor and Decker 2008) But it is also up to those that bring about these revolutionary changes to not allow them to become a distortion from whence they came. What we "see" as fact is determined by the organizing idea; if we change the organizing idea - the paradigm - we can then "see" something different. (Verspoor and Decker 2008) "The power of the organising idea is such that it can discover things which are not yet seen by many others, and indeed, which often goes counter to the existing evidence, which is based on the prevailing idea or belief. It is only later, under the impetus of the new organising idea, that nature reveals the evidence to the extent that it becomes accepted." (Verspoor and Decker 2008)

Modern science basically began with Copernicus' discovery that it was the Earth that revolved around the Sun; that it moved and rotated on its own axis. How did he *know* this? In the early part of the 16th century, he certainly did not fly out beyond Earth to witness this, so he had <u>no</u> observational evidence to back up his "discovery" contrary to common thought. In fact, at that time, there was considerable more observational evidence to the contrary; even today there is the inescapable fact that the movement of Earth is contradicted by our immediate senses. (Bortoft 1996) So was this really a "discovery"? There was no scientific method that allowed Copernicus to immediately see this phenomenon. Indeed, his discovery was a gradual acceptance to the point that by the time there actually was observational confirmation of his heliocentric universe theory in 1838, it was almost superfluous. (Bortoft 1996) But yet, this was unarguably one of the major "revolutions" within science. But what facilitated, what motivated Copernicus to adopt this completely, at that time, radical organizing idea? The concept of wholeness. What he saw in the current mathematical model that said that everything revolved around Earth was a lack of harmony, a lack of unity. (Verspoor and Decker 2008) and (Bortoft 1996)

How does this apply to equine nutrition? It's simple…we must view the horse through the looking glass of holistic science so as to arrive at the undistorted organizing idea of what is an appropriate diet. With everything we have discussed in the foregoing, it would be a complete ignorance of the science to arrive at any other conclusion than a biologically appropriate diet that honors the horse's integrative functions (and I include in this not just the physical, but the etheric and astral bodies). From what we've seen throughout this book, there is no nutrient factor that a horse cannot obtain via a diet of organic foraging … *if* the soil supports the growth of healthy organic plant material. This also does not mean a monoculture pasture, which would equate to not much more than force feeding. If the horse is being "used" in such a way as to grossly exceed his nutrient requirements to the point he has to be sustained with artificial foods, then there is an issue to be dealt with that lies outside the field of equine nutrition.

As I mentioned in the Minerals section, the following is a discussion on Calcium & Silicon, just for reading purposes. [It is not intended it to be a "testing" component if you are taking this as part of the A.C.A.N. certification course.]

6.2   Calcium & Silicon

There is an issue that is generating some discussion in human nutrition as it may play into equine nutrition as well. That is the issue of calcium and silicon and the ability of the latter to *transmute* into the former in the body. There seems to be a dominant view in the medical field, even among many "holistic" practitioners, that supplemental (mineral) calcium can replace bone calcium (that which can be detected as Ca via lab analysis), especially in aging women and regarding the issue of osteoporosis. This in turn can be correlated to horses with regard to various pathologies relating to both hard (bone) tissue and connective tissue as well as normal remodeling. The primary difference between conventional and "alternative" recommendations with regard to calcium supplementation appears to lie mainly with the issue of absorption, the latter group many times stating that "bioactive" minerals are much better absorbed by the body. That statement alone has much truth to it, however some evidence may indicate that we are not actually using the correct mineral by attempting to replace bone calcium with supplementation of mineral calcium. I am not really stating any position here, but instead offering the reader something to explore further if so desired; this can involve a basic understanding of minerals relative to the works of individuals such as Rudolf Steiner and Harvey Lisle, and particularly C. Louis Kervran for the purpose of this discussion. As I have stated previously, we should be looking at the physiological evolutionary requirements to lead us in the direction of a species appropriate feeding regimen for horses; as well, we should not ignore the *behavioral* feeding aspects of the free-ranging horse. Dr. William R. Jackson, PhD, is at least one research scientist that has reached the conclusion that supplemental mineral calcium has the potential to cause more harm than good (again, speaking of the human realm). His assertion is that affected individuals (those suffering bone loss) who take calcium supplements are then suffering other signs such as decaying teeth, brittle bones, and other signs of calcium discomfort and dissipation. (Jackson 2004) He goes on to say that "Not only does this form of calcium [my note: he is referring to supplemental mineral calcium] fail to restore calcium deficiency, but it also may cause extensive and painful damage." (Jackson 2004) The body cannot eliminate excess or unusable calcium and reacts to protect vital organs by recirculating the portion of unusable supplemental calcium and depositing it into joints and non-vital tissues; normal calcium deficiencies then are compounded with calcified joints and tissues [e.g. arthritis]. (Jackson 2004) He further states that sclerosed arteries contain 140% less silica than do normal arteries; and silica always disappears from bones that are becoming osteoporotic.

Lack of silicon in the diets of laboratory animals almost always results in bone and cartilage deformation. (Jackson 2004) And as we saw above, silicon is the second most abundant element on Earth at just under 30% (silicon and oxygen together make up ~75% of the Earth's crust). One must wonder why it is so plentiful if it has no significant dietary use. If it is dietary silica that is needed much more than dietary calcium, how does the calcium get in the body, and how does the body derive the benefits of calcium? Professor Louis C. Kervran, a former Minister of Health in France, has demonstrated that silica transmutes into calcium. "Assisted by official laboratories in France, Kervran and associates concluded that the calcium needed by animal cells seldom is derived from mineral calcium; rather, it is the product of "biological transmutations" from silica and other elements." (Jackson 2004) [Quotes original] It is well known that siliceous rocks become calcareous through the actions of micro-organisms; the plant horsetail (Equisetum) which is rich in silica, was used for recalcification in ancient times. (Kervran *et al.* 1998) Prof. Kervran further states that mineral calcium is a residue and is not assimilated by the organism: "In man and higher animals it exists in a terminal form, but plants and micro-organisms carry out the reverse reaction and utilise calcium." (Kervran *et al.* 1998) Could this be a reason we so often see calcium in horse's urine? According to Kervran, for recalcification to occur, conditions must be established for the organism (man and higher animals) to *manufacture its own calcium*, primarily through plant-based silica. He further states that silica in its elemental form (i.e., that not taken up by plants per Kervran) has a contrary, or *decalcifying* effect. (Kervran *et al.* 1998) [emphasis mine] A research experiment demonstrated that chickens deprived of calcium produced soft-shelled eggs, yet when fed mica, which contains potassium and silica but not calcium, the ability to lay calcium-rich, hard-shelled eggs was restored, indicating an ability to biologically transmute potassium and silica into calcium. These same researchers performed another controlled experiment regarding animals with broken bones: vegetal silica was given to animals in one group while the control group was not allowed vegetal silica but was fed mineral calcium. The group fed vegetal silica had bones that healed quicker and stronger than the control group. (Jackson 2004) Yet another study published in the (human) Journal of Nutritional Health and Aging states that: "Accumulating evidence over the last 30 years strongly suggest that dietary silicon is beneficial to bone and connective tissue health and we recently reported strong positive associations between dietary Si intake and bone mineral density in US and UK cohorts." (Jugdaohsingh 2007) In horses, it has been observed that silicon facilitates (acts as a catalyst in) the formation of collagen and bone mineralization, although the mechanism is still unknown. (Gill 2009) What Prof. Kervran said regarding plant-based minerals vs their elemental form is a vital key to mineral nutrition for animals (and humans). Beach sand is rich in silica but cannot be used as a supplement until it is assimilated by plant life. But Prof. Kervran was also careful to note that the plant must be utilized *during its growth stage*, what we might think of as the "digestive" stage; mature plants set mineral silica and is useless and can be harmful inasmuch as it can actually cause decalcification. During the growth stage, the animal will not only ingest silica but all the associative enzymes, hormones and other bio-factors. (Jackson 2004) As we have previously seen, pasture grasses, especially those of the C4 variety are rich in silica.

The subject of biological transmutation is debated and many scientists do not agree that it is possible; some who have tried to replicate the so-called "Kervran Effect" have not been successful. Orthodox biochemical science has had the axiom [or should I say, verisimilitude?] of "in a chemical reaction, matter is neither created nor destroyed" basically since its inception by Lavoisier in the 18th century; in other words nothing chemically can change short of a "hot" nuclear reaction. Then cold fusion appeared on the scene in 1989, which of course many scientists today still refute its possibility. Goethe is often quoted as saying: "One perceives the fundamental essence of life in the living, not the inanimate, in that which is changing, not what is finished." Kervran said: "It is evident that biological chemistry is mistaken in trying, exclusively, to apply chemical analyses to the study of living matter. When a molecule is taken away from a living cell it is impossible to study the cell's properties. The latter are dependent on the position of the molecule in a component and on the coupling of these components which, together, give rise to the many interactions characteristic of life." (Kervran *et al.* 1998)

In a 2000 review of Dr. Kervran's book, *Biological Transmutations*, Dr. Eugene Mallove had this to say (Source: http://www.infinite-energy.com/iemagazine/issue34/bookreview_biotrans.html):

"Reading this translation and compilation of a number of Prof. Louis Kervran's pre-1970 works is very disturbing, producing the disorientation that accompanies a possible deep paradigm shift in science. Kervran (1901-1983), a medical scientist and engineer with a high official position in the French research and occupational health community, had a life-long interest in the possibility of biological transmutations. His curiosity apparently began in his youth when he watched the hens pecking at specks of mica in the farmyard. His later professional observations concerned (in one small part) the anomalous re-appearance of robust calcium-bearing eggshells in calcium-deprived chickens that had been administered dietary mica (a potassium-rich mineral). Over a century earlier (in 1799), French chemist Louis Nicolas Vauquelin had noted this. The Kervran bio-transmutation story and its background is summarized eloquently in "Alchemists in the Garden," a chapter of the best-selling book The Secret Life of Plants by Peter Tompkins and the late Christopher Bird.

If Kervran's thesis is true, how could mainstream researchers, through the era of sophisticated modern biochemistry and molecular biology, have missed the omnipresence of biological nuclear transmutation? The critics' answer is simple: biological transmutation is delusion or fabrication—just as cold fusion remains, from their perspective. Post-1989 cold fusion critics, in fact, used the Kervran story to mock Fleischmann and Pons by linking them with a man they said believed in "nuclear powered chickens." But for those who seriously examine the evidence for inorganic, low-energy nuclear reactions and heavy element transmutation on electrodes in cold fusion experiments, there is sufficient reason to take Kervran's hypothesis seriously. If non-biological low-energy nuclear reactions (LENR) exist in the laboratory, why not in the natural world?

Indeed, with the backdrop of the cold fusion/LENR experience of the past eleven years, Kervran's work acquires far more significance. It may well turn out that cold fusion studies, pregnant as they are with revolutionary science and technology, may be but a late-blossoming appendage to a much greater truth about what Mother Nature herself has developed. This possibility may offend some cold fusion investigators, who perhaps fancy that they "got there first." We know how uncomfortable some cold fusion researchers are with the copious evidence for heavy element transmutation in modern experiments. Eventually it may be recognized that pioneers, such as Prof. Kervran, were on the low-energy nuclear reaction pathway long before the Utah announcement.

Kervran's thesis is that the transmutation of elements, in particular by reactions among the first few dozen of the periodic table, occurs regularly in biological systems—both in microbes and in multicellular organisms such as human beings. Transmutation is inherent to biology. He concluded that hydrogen and oxygen nuclei primarily, by adding or subtracting from other nuclei, is the essence of transmutation in biology. Some examples: $11Na + 8O$ --> $19K$; $19K + 1H$ --> $20Ca$; $20Ca - 1H$ --> $19K$; or $12Mg + 8O$ --> $20Ca$. Carbon might also participate, e.g. $14Si + 6C$ --> $20Ca$. Kervran did not suggest how such exothermic and endothermic bio-nuclear reactions might be facilitated at the nuclear-atomic level (others would do that later1), but he did collect and correlate many anomalous biochemical observations from nineteenth and twentieth century researchers. He claimed these supported his conclusions, but he also made original observations and conducted his own experiments. If Kervran's thesis is correct, the natural world may teem with countless bio-alchemical factories, which, in turn, work profound alterations in the mineralogical composition of the planet. Geophysics Prof. M. Camberfort wrote to Kervran in 1974, "I have spoken of your work in my most recent book, because I consider that your hypotheses, largely confirmed in certain cases, are the only ones susceptible of explaining a number of facts noted by geologists, so far explained (in geological circles) by fairy tales and old wives' tales." Astronomer Carl Sagan, on the other hand, wrote to Kervran in 1962: "The types of reactions which you are proposing are quite impossible in ordinary chemistry. . .I would strongly suggest that you read an elementary textbook in nuclear physics." Sagan died in 1996, never having come to terms with cold fusion or Kervran.

In papers and books from 1959 through 1983, Kervran synthesized his biotransmutation ideas. Notable among his books, all published by Librarie Maloine in France , are: Biological Transmutations (1962), Proofs in Geology and Physics of Weak Energy Transmutations (1973), Proofs in Biology of Weak Energy Transmutation (1975), and Biological Transmutations and Modern Physics (1983). For the softbound English edition under review, translator Michel Abehsera compiled and adapted an apparently small but representative portion of Kervran's work prior to 1970. In his Foreword, Abehsera describes a meeting with Kervran: ". . .he showed himself such a dragon in science that nothing but science was discussed. . .he knew his subject well; he seemed to have read all the scientific books and articles published all over the world, to know the work of every living scientist. And when I told him that he had given to science a new direction and hope, he answered, his face growing red, 'I simply pointed out what has always existed.'"

During his lifetime Kervran received support for his work from several mainstream scientists who conducted biotransmutation experiments. Prominent among these was Prof. Pierre Baranger, chief of the Laboratory for Organic Chemistry at the École

Polytechnique in Paris. Prof. Baranger in the late 1950s repeated the seed growth experiments of von Herzeele (conducted and published from 1876 to 1883), in which elements appeared to be produced in seeds sprouted in distilled water alone (based on analysis of the ashed seeds and plants). Von Herzeele had found that phosphorus went to sulfur, calcium to phosphorus, magnesium into calcium, etc.—many of the findings that Kervran would later ratify. Baranger reported his work in January 1958 at a prestigious scientific institute in Switzerland. In an interview with the magazine Science et Vie in 1959,2 he said:

My results look impossible, but there they are. I have taken every precaution. I have repeated the experiments many times. I have made thousands of analyses for years. I have had the results verified by third parties who did not know what I was about. I have used several different methods. I changed my experimenters. But there is no way out; we have to submit to the evidence: plants know the old secret of the alchemists. Every day under our very gaze they are transmuting elements. . .I have been teaching chemistry at the École Polytechnique for twenty years, and believe me, the laboratory which I direct is no den of false science. But I have never confused respect for science with the taboos imposed by intellectual conformism. For me, any meticulously performed experiment is a homage to science even if it shocks our ingrained habits. Von Herzeele's experiments were too few to be absolutely convincing. But their results inspired me to control them with all the precaution possible in a modern lab and to repeat them enough times so that they would be statistically irrefutable. That's what I've done.

No matter how solid the experimental evidence, biological transmutation, like cold fusion and inorganic low-energy transmutation, flies in the face of a paradigm that began at the very foundation of chemistry in the late eighteenth century: elements retain their identities—they do not change into other elements. Antoine Laurent Lavoisier (1743-1794), widely considered to be the "father of chemistry" or even the "Newton of chemistry," according to Isaac Asimov,[3] is responsible for that paradigm. We may regard this as a brilliant insight that was perhaps necessary to help make sense of the bewildering facts that emerged from centuries of alchemical experimentation. Moreover, the paradigm is ordinarily true, but the problem with the dogma launched by Lavoisier (ironically at the very time his contemporary Vauquelin was questioning the origin of calcium in chicken egg shells!) is that it has been too powerful, too rigid, and too enduring.

Lavoisier's scientific career ended on May 8, 1794, when he was guillotined during the French Revolution for having ties to "tax farmers."[3] His paradigm of element immutability survived the discovery of radioactivity in 1896 and the host of other conventionally accepted nuclear reactions. Unfortunately, it has grown so strong over two centuries that resistance to cold fusion, low-energy nuclear reactions, and especially biological transmutation remains intense. However, prior to the explosion of biochemical knowledge in the mid to late twentieth century at least one significant voice was raised in support of greater circumspection. Louis de Broglie, one of the luminaries of modern quantum mechanics is quoted by Kervran: "It is premature to reduce the vital process to the quite insufficiently developed conceptions of nineteenth and even twentieth century physics and chemistry."

Perhaps it is time to return to the wisdom of de Broglie. Kervran's work may have been a beginning in that direction. This book, though limited in scope and in places lacking the detail that is surely available in Kervran's original material, is a very useful introduction and overview of Kervran's ideas and the field of biological transmutation. This area seems destined to grow, especially with the recent founding of a formal society for the study of bio-transmutation, according to the announcement by French cold fusion researcher Dr. Jean-Paul Biberian.[4] Experimenters from France to Japan are now hard at work on this exciting new frontier. Others have already published contemporary scientific works.5,6,7 We occasionally even hear rumors that certain biotechnology companies may be working in this area!

Though this book includes a six-page bibliography, and footnotes do provide many additional references to the scientific literature, it is disappointing that not all scientific studies referred to by name are adequately referenced. That is a small price to pay for the vista that this book opens on a possible new reality that may have been within us and around us for so long. The potential implications for science, technology, agriculture, and medicine are so large, the work of Kervran and of those who came before him demands great attention and the most thorough investigation."

Dr. Eugene Mallove, founder of Infinite Energy magazine, the New Energy Foundation, and one of a group of scientists that tirelessly fought for the acceptance of the cold fusion theory and thus an abundance of clean, safe, low-cost energy for the world, was murdered on May 14, 2004.

The implication of biological transmutation within equine nutrition is no less important than it is in human nutrition; the ramifications of the possibility of mineral transmutation of course affects forced crude mineral supplementation and the potential to create imbalances.

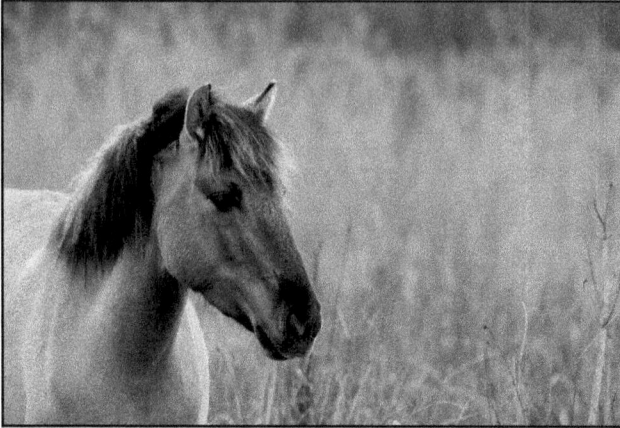

Figure 23: Konik horse
Shutterstock.com image # 101301949 © Davy Veelaert

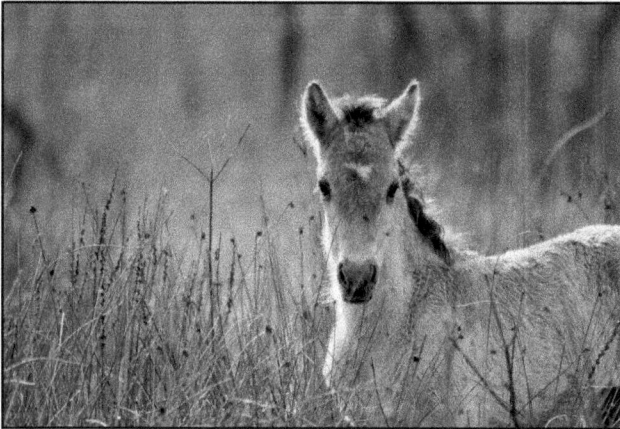

Figure 24: Konik foal
Shutterstock.com image # 101301952 © Davy Veelaert

A rare breed of horse has been recognized as a key part of plans to restore delicate wetlands. It is now acknowledged that the grazing habits of the rare Konik breed – the name meaning small horse in Polish – play a crucial part in helping to make wetlands more habitable for other species. They are a highly unusual breed, descended directly from the Tarpan, the wild European forest horse hunted to extinction in Britain in Neolithic times. Tarpan survived in central Europe until the late 1800s when the last were captured in the primeval forest of Bialoweiza, Poland, and taken to zoos. The last died in 1910.

In the early 20th century, Polish scientists noticed Tarpan-colored foals – mouse grey overall with zebra stripes on their legs and dark manes and tails – were still being born to domestic mares in herds where Tarpan had formerly ranged. It was also noticed that they turned whiter over winter – another Tarpan trait. They selected these and back-bred them successfully over generations to recreate the extinct forest horse. Between the two world wars, German zoo directors were supported by senior Nazi party officials such as Herman Goering in their effort to recreate these primeval horses. The Tarpan featured heavily in German folklore and their recreation through racially selective back breeding supported the Nazis eugenic race theories. After the Nazi invasion of Poland, whole herds where stolen and transported back to Germany where matters took a darker turn, the horses becoming part of genetic experiments trying to back-breed a German Tarpan. The horses were sadly eaten by the starving population of Berlin and Munich when the Russians invaded in the final days of the war. Polish scientists looking after wild horse herds managed to protect some, and after the war the protected herds were allowed to repopulate the national parks of Poland under Soviet occupation. When the Iron Curtain fell, conservationists were at last able to transport the wild horses to national parks across Europe.

Wildwood Trust pioneered the introduction of these horses to Britain in 2002. It brought the first ever of their breed to arrive in southern England and these horses and their offspring have been helping to restore some of the most precious national nature reserves in the UK. Since this time, conservation grazing projects throughout Europe have used the Konik horses for wetland grazing projects. The former habitat of Tarpan was marshy woodland where their grazing activities help create ideal living conditions for a host of associated wildlife such as rare geese, spoonbills, bitterns and corncrakes. The project using the Konik to restore the Kentish wetlands is a joint venture between the Wildwood Trust, near Canterbury, English Nature and Kent Wildlife Trust. At present, most of the trust's herd is grazing at nature reserves around the county. Wildwood Trust runs Woodland Discovery Park, a visitor attraction which forms part of their strategy to save native and once-native wildlife from extinction. Its plans involve releasing large wild herbivores and developing conservation grazing systems to restore natural ecological processes to help Britain team with wildlife again. Wildwood includes a forest enclosure where Konik horses retired from the trust's main herds can spend their days, providing the many visitors with a good look at the remarkable breed.

[The above story is edited from an online article titled: *Rare horse breed proves crucial to delicate ecosystem* in Horsetalk.co.nz on Jun 01, 2012 in Horse Breeds.]

APPENDIX I -
TIMELINE OF EQUINE FEEDS
(Carter 2004) - except as noted

1834 - First supplement - Thomas Day, of Day & Sons, starts manufacturing supplements. The equine tonic 'Black drink' costs 10 shillings per half-dozen bottles.

1894 – Ralston Purina develops a horse feed that is "cheaper than oats and safer than corn". (Nestle Purina n.d.)

1906 - Nobel Prize-winning biochemist Frederick Hopkins suggests the existence of vitamins in the human body. In 1912 he publishes a key paper on the subject. This knowledge proves vital in the fields of human and veterinary nutrition.

1907 - Nobel Prize-winning immunologist Elie Metchnikoff introduces the concept of probiotics to benefit humans. These live microbes will later prove popular in animal nutrition.

1920 - Early experimentation begins on the effectiveness of feeding yeast culture to livestock, although equine trials are not carried out for another 60 years.

1929 - The Equivite trademark is registered and its vitamin and mineral mix for horses is launched.

1935 - The first cod liver oil product for horses and ponies is launched, Super Solvitax Pure Cod Liver Oil.

1958 - First pony nuts - The first compound feed for horses, SPILLERS Horse and Pony Cubes is launched.

1960 - The first compound feed for racehorses, SPILLERS Racehorse Cubes, is introduced, followed in 1961 by the first compound feed for broodmares and young stock, SPILLERS Stud Cubes.

1977 - A dust-free, fermented, bagged-forage product providing optimum protein and energy levels is launched in England, HorseHage Ryegrass.

1977 - The first bagged, chopped-fibre feed is introduced by Youngs Animal Feeds, Super Molichop Original.

1978 - The first extruded horse feed is launched by Badminton Specialty Feeds, Triple Crown Extruform. (Extruding involves cooking different feed elements together at high temperatures and reforming them.)

Late 1970s - Micronising, a rapid-cooking process using infra-red heat that increases the digestibility of starch, is pioneered by Dodson & Horrell. Subsequently, one of the first micronized cereal and oat diets, Microfeed, is launched.

1982 - The use of reprocessed bread is pioneered with Baileys' No.1 Cooked Cereal Meal. Bread was the precursor of micronized wheat.

1983 - The yeast culture Yea-Sacc1026 is introduced by biotechnology company Alltech, founded three years earlier.

1984 – Triple Crown Nutrition, Inc. formed in Wisconsin USA. (Triple Crown Nutrition Inc n.d.)

1986 - First herbal calmer - The first herbal calmer for horses is launched, Feedmark's Steady Up.

1987 – The Chaffhaye Company was founded in Dell City, TX, making the first 50# bag "haylage" product in the US, thus solving the problem of spoilage typical of on-farm produced haylage or silage. It is a chopped, fermented pasture product of either alfalfa or Bermuda grass. (Chaffhaye Inc. n.d.)

1989 - First balancer - The first feed balancer is launched under the provisional name of Gro-Well Equine Feed Balancer, before changing to Equilibra. The pelleted feed contains vitamins, minerals, proteins and yeast and is said to improve feed utilization.

1989 - The first 'flash-dried' alfalfa chop, Alfa A (now called Alfa-A Original), is introduced to the UK market by Dengie, and high-temperature-dried alfalfa is hailed as 'the introduction of forage feeds'.

1989 - The first balancer formulated specifically for breeding stock is developed by Baileys Horse Feeds. It allows for the feeding of a low-starch diet.

Late 1980s - A revolutionary muesli diet for the leisure horse is introduced by Dodson & Horrell, Pasture Mix. The product is also one of the first horse feeds to contain herbs.

1990 - Following this year's World Equestrian Games, extensive research is carried out on exercising horses in extreme heat by Kentucky Equine Research.

1990 - First for feet - The first complex formula to support hoof growth and health is launched by NAF, Hoof and Hide supplement.

1990 - Alltech launches bio-available [the extent to which a nutrient can be used by the body] organic minerals easily absorbed in the gut, Bioplex Trace Minerals.

1991 - First veteran feed - The first pellet-free muesli mix for the older horse, Allen & Page's Old Faithful's Special Blend, is launched.

1992 - Robert Eustace FRCVS, who sits on the scientific committee of the Laminitis Trust, highlights the link between obesity and laminitis, publishing the paper Explaining Laminitis and its Prevention.

1993 – Tri-Forage Farms Ltd is formed in Bath, ON, Canada. The company markets a variety of different long-stem grass and/or alfalfa hays that are bagged and fermented (haylage). (Triforage Horsehae n.d.)

1994 - First for laminitis - The first low-sugar/starch feed for animals prone to laminitis is developed by Dengie. Hi-Fi Lite is the first product to carry the Laminitis Trust Approval (the trust launches its feed approval mark seven years later).

APPENDIX 2 -
GMOs, Glyphosate & Tomorrow

By Don Huber, PhD

REPRINTED WITH PERMISSION

To view this on the web,
please see http://farmandranchfreedom.org/sff/Huber-May2011-Acres.pdf

INTERVIEW

GMOs, Glyphosate & Tomorrow

Distinguished Professor, Scientist Reveals Growing, Multi-Faceted
Problems in Glyphosate & Crops Created to Survive It

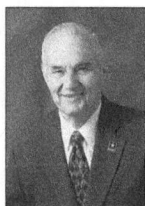

**Don
Huber, Ph.D.**

Seeds evolved for millions of years before humans invented corporate agribusiness. Genetic selection to improve crops began only when people invented farming. Early on, there was a vast germ pool from which to select differences in vigor, growth, quality characteristics, yield or disease resistance. Even after years of extensive selection and later blending into hybrids by diligent researchers during the past century, most of this inheritance is unpatentable and therefore useless as a source of power or corporate-style profit.

Genetic engineering to modify crops exists because most of the world's farmers depend on seeds, and as a novel way to manipulate genes it offered inviolate proprietary control. Two traits account for practically all of the genetically modified crops grown in the world today. One deploys herbicide-tolerance enabled by a glyphosate-insensitive form of the EPSPS gene coding (key to this GMO is the soil bacterium Agrobacterium tumefaciens). The other uses insect-resistance due to one or more toxin genes derived from the soil bacterium Bacillus thuringiensis.

It is the former that concerns us here, for without glyphosate, the biotech industry would be an orphan, all dressed up with nowhere to go. Glyphosate, often known as Roundup® after the popular Monsanto product but available in many guises since its patent expired in 2000, is the partner GMOs must bring to the dance. It is a broad-spectrum herbicide that ingeniously ties up nutrient access rather than killing unwanted plants directly. It was heralded for many years as a relatively benign replacement for the horrific, dioxin-based herbicides of the past. The figures don't lie; GMOs drive glyphosate sales.

Enter Don Huber, a plant pathologist of 50 years standing, now Emeritus Professor at Purdue University and enjoying an active post-academic life. Huber is an international authority on nutrient deficiency diseases of plants and is particularly well situated to comment on glyphosate as it functions through nutrient tie-up, not inherent toxicity.

Recently his retirement turned hyperactive when a letter he wrote to Secretary of Agriculture Tom Vilsack leaked out. Although much of the mainstream media ignored it, the letter was an immediate sensation. Huber — not coincidentally a speaker at the 2010 Acres U.S.A. Conference — informed Vilsack that a new infectious agent had been discovered. It is "widespread, very serious, and in much higher concentrations in Roundup Ready (RR) soybeans and corn," he wrote. He appealed to the secretary for help with resources and research capability.

The letter unleashed a storm of alarm and denial, and as Huber tells below, the USDA is looking into the matter despite its recent ill-advised approval of genetically modified alfalfa.

We asked him to comment on his recent letter (see pages 54-55) and share his own thoughts and opinions on this ubiquitous farm chemical.

— Chris Walters

ACRES U.S.A. How does glyphosate differ from herbicides that were popular before it came along?

DON HUBER. There are a number of ways that glyphosate is different from most other herbicides. Most of our herbicides are mineral chelators that act to physiologically immobilize a specific mineral nutrient that is required for a specific critical enzyme. When that physiological pathway is shut down, the weed or the plant it's applied to dies. Glyphosate also is a chemical chelator that can grab onto mineral nutrients and immobilize them physiologically so they're no longer available for those physiologic functions that they regulate. The difference with glyphosate is that it is not specific to just one mineral nutrient, but immobilizes many of them and doesn't affect a primary mechanism to cause death by itself. It merely turns off the plant's defense mechanisms so that soil-borne fungi that would normally take weeks to months to damage a plant can kill it in just a few days after glyphosate is applied. When they use the glyphosate-tolerant technology, they insert another gene that keeps that plant's defense mechanism going somewhat so you can put the glyphosate directly on the crop plant without having it killed. But the technology doesn't do anything to the glyphosate, which is still tying up mineral nutrients. Anytime you put the gene in, you reduce the nutrient efficiency of the plant, though not to the point that it destroys the ability of the plant to survive. It does leave it physiologically impaired.

ACRES U.S.A. Before glyphosate-tolerant genes were introduced, how did farmers cope with the danger of possibly killing the crop plant?

HUBER. They took care of their weed control before planting or before the crop emerged. Back then, there weren't too many herbicides that you could apply directly to the plant. We had a few, 2,4-D and a few others, that were semi-selective and very effective against broadleaves, which have a different physiology than grass plants. A similar thing with Tordon. You can put Tordon right on a grass pasture and it will kill the

broadleaf weeds for three or four years. It has pretty good residual activity, but grass looks like you'd just fertilized it when you got rid of all of those broadleaved weeds.

ACRES U.S.A. The innovation that gave glyphosate its market clout had to do with concentrating the whole arsenal into one weapon? No more multiple herbicides?

be. In a high-clay soil it may survive for a number of years. In water solution it can degrade fairly rapidly and not have a lot of residual activity. I think that's probably one reason why the French Supreme Court ruled two years ago that it would be fraud to claim biodegradability of glyphosate in soil — because it's not always really predictable. For some soils it can survive for a long period of time, and in others it may have a much shorter period. With the information that's cur-

> "Any time you have a single gene in so many different crops, especially a gene that impacts the normal resistance and defense mechanism in the plant, and you spread that same vulnerability across so many plants, you should anticipate a high level of vulnerability."

HUBER. There was selective activity in our herbicides. Glyphosate on plants without the new gene inserted has a very broad-spectrum effect so that all weeds are affected. They're all killed by the soil fungi. It's not quite analogous, but you could say that what you're doing with glyphosate is you're giving the plant a bad case of AIDS. You've shut down the immune system or the defense system.

ACRES U.S.A. How does glyphosate's immobility as a strong metal chelator or nutrient chelator translate into the long-term effects of glyphosate buildup after years of steady use?

HUBER. As long as it's bound very tightly with those mineral elements it is not available or not in an active form for plant damage. If there is something that happens to break that binding then it can again be released and available for root uptake and plant damage. It depends on how long it survives in the soil and that will depend on two primary factors. Soil pH is a big factor in stability and the other is clay content. The higher the pH, the less stable it is, and the higher the clay content, the more stable it will

rently available, it's not really possible to have a good predictable figure. We do know that even though it's immobilized rapidly in most soils it can then be reactivated or desorbed and reactivated to damage future crops.

ACRES U.S.A. What must happen to reactivate it?

HUBER. One of the things that's recently been shown to do this is to apply phosphorus fertilizer on the crop. From a nutritional standpoint, it can actually desorb the glyphosate so that it's again reactivated as an active chemical for plant uptake and damage.

ACRES U.S.A. Has this been demonstrated by researchers to impact the crops when it's desorbed?

HUBER. Yes. That can be quite damaging to the crop and actually limit uptake of nutrients required by the crop as much as 60 to 70 percent, and that's pretty much across the board. Most elements will be reduced around 60 percent and a few of them in the 70 percent range. In this way the plant can be placed under a

INTERVIEW

fairly significant nutrient deficiency even though the nutrients may be in the soil — the plant can't utilize them because of glyphosate's toxicity.

ACRES U.S.A. Have your colleagues found similar impacts?

HUBER. Yes. A number of soil microbiologists are all reporting the same type of impact on the soil biology. One paper mentions that it's a very powerful herbicide, but also a very potent biocide. It's a little bit selective in that it stimulates some soil organisms and is very toxic

> ## "It's not quite analogous, but you could say that what you're doing with glyphosate is you're giving the plant a bad case of AIDS. You've shut down the immune system or the defense system."

to other organisms. It's toxic to your legume module bacteria for nitrogen fixation, also quite toxic to the organisms that make manganese and iron available for plant uptake, and those are critical nutrients. It stimulates the soil pathogens that do the killing from a weed control standpoint, but it also stimulates some so that you're essentially making a super-pathogen to kill a weed. Then you leave that super-pathogen in the soil, which also attacks other plants later on in the rotation.

ACRES U.S.A. The letter you sent to Secretary of Agriculture Tom Vilsack in January, not surprisingly, is being attacked on a number of fronts. Since the pathogen that has been discovered hasn't been detailed in a journal, its existence has been questioned. How was this pathogen discovered, who did the research, and is research being readied for publication?

HUBER. The letter to the Secretary wasn't for public dissemination. It was a request for help. It was meant to bring to his attention the things that many of us are seeing out in the field, both from the veterinarians and animal producers as well as agronomists, plant patholo-

gists and our crop producers. I wanted to bring the situation to his attention and request help so we could move the science along faster than we can individually. It's because of the seriousness of the situation that many growers are experiencing. The work to date has been very well done, very scientifically conducted, but there is still much to do. Much of it hasn't been published on the animal side, but Koch's-postulates — the scientific criteria used to establish a cause-effect relationship — have been completed, and much of the science on the animal side has been done. That's not a concern or a question. The veterinarians have been very thorough. They split their samples, sent them to a number of different labs to rule out all of the other known causes of those conditions, and when they check for this new organism that's what they find. They find it with cattle and pigs and horses and poultry. So it has a pretty broad host range. In trying to identify how the animals were being infected, they began looking at the feed and found that soybean meal was just loaded with it. They also find it in silage and corn products. Any fermented product seems to encourage this organism. It's also a very good synergist with other pathogens. The Fusarium fungus that causes Sudden Death Syndrome (SDS) is very compatible with this new organism. Another interesting thing is that it appears very compatible with Clavibacter that causes Goss' wilt of corn as well as other bacteria. Over the past two years we've had extensive SDS and Goss' wilt epidemics and that's where we really see the higher titer with this organism. The two diseases and the newly discovered pathogen appear to be very synergistic. This new organism may be an opportunist that is able to take advantage of a weakened condition and then really move forward.

ACRES U.S.A. What is "higher titer?"

HUBER. Higher population. Just a lot more of it. It seems to grow better for possibly a higher infection potential.

ACRES U.S.A. Is this the first appearance of this pathogen in nature? Or is it something that was there all along, waiting for discovery?

HUBER. We're fairly convinced it's something that's always been there, very benign, not really a problem until we changed something that has either increased its virulence or its opportunity. I think the research to date would indicate that it's probably more a change in the susceptibility of the crops, in the population of the pathogen, and in the potential for animal infection. There are many organisms new to science that have been around forever. Which is something you see with the prions. We didn't know they existed either until we had to look a lot further to find an answer to a problem, and then they were discovered. This organism was discovered pretty much the same way. When they rule out all other known sources, then the veterinarians just kept looking and found this one, and then verified it as the cause by doing Koch's postulates. Then they took it a step further to find out: where was it coming from? How are the animals getting it? That led them to check the feed and they found it there. In science you go from one thing to another, sometimes in a process, and you don't necessarily stop and publish each little bit that is found until you have a better understanding of how it all fits together. In agriculture we're really talking about a system; we're not talking about silver bullets.

ACRES U.S.A. People have an easier time understanding single-factor analysis and silver bullets, but that's not how it works in nature, is it?

HUBER. We're talking about how parts of this system interact and fit together. That's been the real emphasis in this research, not how to get that publicity and meet the popular demand by publishing each little bit of information. You try to get enough research so you can really understand its scope and what its impact is in the overall production system. That's really my plea to the Secretary in that letter — we need resources and we need some commitment of those resources and personnel that are available to the Secretary but aren't available to each individual scientist. It was for alerting him to the problem so he would be interested, as he has been, in passing it on to those who would be able to provide additional resources. We need to understand how it fits into the overall ecological scheme and agricultural production system.

ACRES U.S.A. Despite the recent rapid approval of genetically modified alfalfa, do you find a silver lining in indications that USDA resources or commitment are forthcoming?

HUBER. Well, I certainly hope so.

ACRES U.S.A. This pathogen doesn't have a name. What do you call it?

HUBER. That's been a bit of a stumbling block. In the letter I called it a microfungus. That was a mistake, because when you think of a microfungus you automatically think of a mold-type organism, and it certainly isn't that. It's many thousands of times smaller than a mold, much smaller than a bacterium — approximately the size of a virus. It's in that category, except that it self-replicates and can be passive.

ACRES U.S.A. But it is certainly not a virus.

HUBER. Not by our current definition.

ACRES U.S.A. Could your theory be summarized thusly — this is not the result of a mutation in an existing pathogen, rather, a change in the conditions has caused an existing pathogen to multiply and become a problem, with pathways being created that were not common in the past?

HUBER. Right. The organism appears to be prominent in the environment but new to science. On a much larger scale, it would be like when they bred the Texas male-sterile gene into corn. We got away with it for a few years. Then all of a

sudden we realized we had an organism out there that was new to science with the Southern corn leaf blight epidemic of 1970-71. We'd previously had that experience with the Victoria gene in oats.

ACRES U.S.A. Can you name some of the researchers who are involved? Specifically who discovered the pathogen?

HUBER. No. Because there's no need for them to have the harassment or be inundated the way I've been. We've got too much work to do.

ACRES U.S.A. But you can vouch for them?

HUBER. They are very well-established scientists. There's no need to attack everybody else, and that's exactly what happens when you come up with something that's new.

ACRES U.S.A. In other words, naysayers are assured that there is more than one person involved with this research, they're reputable people, the results are going to be published as soon as they're available, and these plant and animal afflictions are not going away?

HUBER. Clavibacter survives in corn residue for three to four years at least so if we continue to do the same things, we should anticipate the same result. There's research that shows that when you apply formulated glyphosate to a glyphosate-tolerant corn plant that normally is resistant, some hybrids become fully susceptible to that organism. Glyphosate can nullify the genetic resistance for Clavibacter just like it can sugar beets for Rhizoctonia or Fusarium in same plants.

ACRES U.S.A. What other results do you anticipate?

HUBER. High infertility and abortions in animals fed with corn and soybean feeds containing high populations of this organism.

ACRES U.S.A. Some of your critics reject the whole idea that sudden plant death and spontaneous cattle abortions are even an increasing problem.

HUBER. It isn't a universal phenomenon, just as most disease outbreaks can be limited. I think the criticism goes against the statistics though. If you look at the USDA's anticipated yield on corn that they put out in August, and then subtract the actual yields reported in January, you come up with almost a billion bushels less, even though we had near ideal conditions for harvest. Where did those billion bushels go? All you have to do to document that there was a short crop last year is look at the price. We're no longer talking about $3 per bushel corn, we're talking about $6 per bushel. That's not from increased ethanol use, that's from a major shortage in the crop produced. How do you get soybeans from $5 up to $12? You have a short crop because you have an inelastic supply/demand relationship in agriculture. I think the figures document that. In some areas they didn't have those problems this year as some had last year, and that's because environmental conditions are also important for disease.

ACRES U.S.A. Just to get it on the record, after you sent your letter to Vilsack, someone else leaked it?

HUBER. Right. It was not intended as a public document. My request to the Secretary was for the help we needed to get resources, and also to ask him to delay any decision on the Roundup Ready alfalfa until some things could be checked out. One reason is that we were seeing a marked increase in susceptibility to Goss' wilt in previously Goss' wilt-resistant corn. Critical research was needed to document the epidemiology of this new organism.

ACRES U.S.A. What has your experience been over the last decade or so with the availability of research funds for questions like this in the United States?

HUBER. Funding for applied research is hard to come by and publishing in this area can also be difficult. I know from the International Symposium on Glyphosate that they had to find a journal publisher outside this country to publish the research data and symposium proceedings. It's pretty hard to get it published in the States. There are also

Letter Sent to Secretary Vilsack by Dr. Huber That Was Leaked

January 16, 2011

Dear Secretary Vilsack:

A team of senior plant and animal scientists have recently brought to my attention the discovery of an electron microscopic pathogen that appears to significantly impact the health of plants, animals, and probably human beings. Based on a review of the data, it is widespread, very serious, and is in much higher concentrations in Roundup Ready (RR) soybeans and corn — suggesting a link with the RR gene or more likely the presence of Roundup. This organism appears NEW to science.

This is highly sensitive information that could result in a collapse of US soy and corn export markets and significant disruption of domestic food and feed supplies. On the other hand, this new organism may already be responsible for significant harm (see below). My colleagues and I are therefore moving our investigation forward with speed and discretion, and seek assistance from the USDA and other entities to identify the pathogen's source, prevalence, implications, and remedies.

We are informing the USDA of our findings at this early stage, specifically due to your pending decision regarding approval of RR alfalfa. Naturally, if either the RR gene or Roundup itself is a promoter or co-factor of this pathogen, then such approval could be a calamity. Based on the current evidence, the only reasonable action at this time would be to delay deregulation at least until sufficient data has exonerated the RR system, if it does.

For the past 40 years, I have been a scientist in the professional and military agencies that evaluate and prepare for natural and manmade biological threats, including germ warfare and disease outbreaks. Based on this experience, I believe the threat we are facing from this pathogen is unique and of a high risk status. In layman's terms, it should be treated as an emergency.

A diverse set of researchers working on this problem have contributed various pieces of the puzzle, which together presents the following disturbing scenario:

Unique Physical Properties

This previously unknown organism is only visible under an electron microscope (36,000X), with an approximate size range equal to a medium size virus. It is able to reproduce and appears to be a micro-fungal-like organism. If so, it would be the first such micro-fungus ever identified. There is strong evidence that this infectious agent promotes diseases of both plants and mammals, which is very rare.

Pathogen Location & Concentration

It is found in high concentrations in Roundup Ready soybean meal and corn, distillers meal, fermentation feed products, pig stomach contents, and pig and cattle placentas.

Linked with Outbreaks of Plant Disease

The organism is prolific in plants infected with two pervasive diseases that are driving down yields and farmer income — sudden death syndrome

continued on next page

some hazards to publishing if you're a young researcher doing research that runs counter to the current popular concepts. A lot of research on safety of genetic engineering is done outside of this country because it's difficult to gain access to the materials, or the statements you have to sign to have access to those materials state that you won't publish without permission of the supplier. I think the 26 entomologists who sent their letter to EPA in 2009 stated it aptly when they said that objective data wasn't available to the EPA because the materials haven't been available to them or that they're denied the opportunity to publish their data.

ACRES U.S.A. Has there been a chilling effect on the availability of funds to do the research in this country?

HUBER. The entomologists asked that they not be publicly identified by name because they were dependent on outside sources for funding and there isn't a lot of funding available for this type of research anymore so that's certainly a major impediment. You have to have funding to get graduate students working on it and if you have the graduate students, then you can get publications out to make it possible for you to get tenure and promotion.

ACRES U.S.A. Is the Ignacio Chapela affair a good example of the impact this can have on a young researcher's career?

HUBER. There are scientists who have experienced a situation where their career became very short or they had to change paths in order to survive and stay in the system.

ACRES U.S.A. Have you received any response from Secretary Vilsack?

HUBER. I didn't anticipate a direct response. I kind of thought I might receive a "We received your letter" note like you get back from your Congressman, but I have been contacted by USDA personnel in response to the letter. I've been cooperating and working with them in that area. I wanted to be able to do that in a more detailed manner than you can put in a letter, so in the letter I merely highlighted the concerns, the things that we were seeing and that we could document. I've been able to provide information for them to go forward in their investigations.

ACRES U.S.A. Then you're confident that the research component of the USDA is looking into it with great interest, not just brushing it aside?

HUBER. I believe they are at this point.

ACRES U.S.A. If the letter had not been made public, if it had gone through channels as you expected, do you think you might have gotten a more proactive response from Vilsack?

HUBER. It might have been easier for him to do that. I don't know. I have a good working relationship with a number of those people in the USDA, and they have the charge to respond to this kind of concern. They can't do it overnight; it takes a little time to get up to speed. Leaking of the letter didn't make it easier for them. It probably made it a little more difficult just because then you get a lot of pressure coming in from all different directions. But it may have moved the process along perhaps a little quicker than it might otherwise.

ACRES U.S.A. Are you personally acquainted with Secretary Vilsack or Assistant Secretary Kathleen Merrigan?

HUBER. No, I'm not. I've worked very closely for a long time with the actual scientists and people doing the work. I have a great deal of respect for a lot of those people.

ACRES U.S.A. What was the major focus of your work during the years before you became a retired, or emeritus, professor?

HUBER. For 50 years my research was focused heavily on the biology and control of soilborne pathogenic fungi, microbial ecology, biological control, microbial interactions and host-parasite physiology — trying to understand resistance and susceptibility from a physiological standpoint. I was heavily involved in the whole development of nitrification inhibitors, and

(SDS) in soy, and Goss' wilt in corn. The pathogen is also found in the fungal causative agent of SDS (Fusarium solani fsp glycines).

Implicated in Animal Reproductive Failure

Laboratory tests have confirmed the presence of this organism in a wide variety of livestock that have experienced spontaneous abortions and infertility. Preliminary results from ongoing research have also been able to reproduce abortions in a clinical setting.

The pathogen may explain the escalating frequency of infertility and spontaneous abortions over the past few years in US cattle, dairy, swine, and horse operations. These include recent reports of infertility rates in dairy heifers of over 20%, and spontaneous abortions in cattle as high as 45%.

For example, 450 of 1,000 pregnant heifers fed wheatlage experienced spontaneous abortions. Over the same period, another 1,000 heifers from the same herd that were raised on hay had no abortions. High concentrations of the pathogen were confirmed on the wheatlage, which likely had been under weed management using glyphosate.

Recommendations

In summary, because of the high titer of this new animal pathogen in Roundup Ready crops, and its association with plant and animal diseases that are reaching epidemic proportions, we request USDA's participation in a multi-agency investigation, and an immediate moratorium on the deregulation of RR crops until the causal/predisposing relationship with glyphosate and/or RR plants can be ruled out as a threat to crop and animal production and human health.

It is urgent to examine whether the side-effects of glyphosate use may have facilitated the growth of this pathogen, or allowed it to cause greater harm to weakened plant and animal hosts. It is well-documented that glyphosate promotes soil pathogens and is already implicated with the increase of more than 40 plant diseases; it dismantles plant defenses by chelating vital nutrients; and it reduces the bioavailability of nutrients in feed, which in turn can cause animal disorders. To properly evaluate these factors, we request access to the relevant USDA data.

I have studied plant pathogens for more than 50 years. We are now seeing an unprecedented trend of increasing plant and animal diseases and disorders. This pathogen may be instrumental to understanding and solving this problem. It deserves immediate attention with significant resources to avoid a general collapse of our critical agricultural infrastructure.

Sincerely,

COL (Ret.) Don M. Huber
Emeritus Professor, Purdue University
APS Coordinator, USDA National Plant Disease Recovery System (NPDRS)

also in identifying nutrient pathways in corn, soybeans and wheat. I served as one of the editors of the American Phytopathological Society's book on mineral nutrition and plant disease, which came out in 2007. I initially got involved with glyphosate thinking that when glyphosate-tolerant soybeans were

released it would probably be a win/win situation for a lot of our growers who didn't want to make a separate trip across the soybeans to meet the nutritional demands for manganese. If they could just add manganese as a tank mix, it would be a pretty good time to remedy the manganese deficiency we

The Basics

Micronutrients are regulators, inhibitors and activators of physiological processes, and plants provide a primary dietary source of these elements for animals and people.

... Lost yield, reduced quality, and increased disease are the unfortunate consequences of untreated micronutrient deficiency. The shift to less tillage, herbicide resistant crops and extensive application of glyphosate has significantly changed nutrient availability and plant efficiency for a number of essential plant nutrients. Some of these changes are through direct toxicity of glyphosate while others are more indirect through changes in soil organisms important for nutrient access, availability, or plant uptake. ...

— From Abstract of "Ag Chemical and Crop Nutrient Interacts Current Update" by Don M. Huber, Emeritus Professor, Purdue University

saw in a number of areas in Indiana, and they could get the weeds controlled at the same time. It only took one trial to realize that it wouldn't work, because glyphosate immobilized the manganese that we were trying to make available for the plant. The last 15-16 years were primarily devoted to understanding and finding ways to remedy the nutrient inefficiency that the technology and the chemistry was imposing on the plant. Of course that brought me right back to looking at a lot of those soil-microbial interactions that are so essential to making nutrients available to plants to start with.

ACRES U.S.A. How does that relate to the current pathogen?

HUBER. Any time you have a single gene in so many different crops, especially a gene that impacts the normal resistance and defense mechanism in the plant, and you spread that same vulnerability across so many plants, you should anticipate a high level of vulnerability. I think that's what we're seeing.

ACRES U.S.A. What worries you about the possibility of this pathogen getting loose in alfalfa?

HUBER. A perennial crop like alfalfa can be very susceptible to a closely related common soilborne bacterium to Goss' wilt. If the technology nullifies resistance to this bacterial disease like it can for corn

and it is compatible with the new organism, then you have a situation where you can compromise the crop totally because you don't have any way to get it out. With an annual crop like corn or soybean, or like we had with the Texas male-sterile gene, it was a matter of just going back to our old genetics and eliminating those with the gene from the breeding program. Once you have it implanted in the plant though, there's no way to get it out. With a perennial, insect-pollinated plant, I don't know of any way to eliminate it once it's distributed throughout an area as it could be very readily.

ACRES U.S.A. Genetic engineering is relatively new to science. Does that bring this problem to a new level of seriousness, because you can't just remove those traits? That is, the way you would if you simply stopped a hybrid program that was making something you didn't like?

HUBER. It's certainly easier to put it in than to get it out. Each time you put a foreign gene in, you're adding another stress to the plant — commonly referred to as a yield-drag aspect, which is very well documented. There's powerful technology here and usually, with a little bit of time, we can find a way to make that work more compatibly. Genetic engineering is a tool we may need for specific situations, but it's also been easy to abuse. I believe that when we start putting all of our eggs in one basket, it increases our vulnerability and potential risk factors

dramatically. I believe we should try to follow scientific principles and use a lot of caution until we understand what's going on in the whole process.

ACRES U.S.A. Do you agree that genetically modified food has been unduly rushed into the American food supply?

HUBER. Someone gave the analogy of asking how many drugs that were on the market 10 years ago aren't on the market today. The reason they aren't on the market now is that new information indicated the side effects were great enough or that they weren't safe for use to start with. Certainly there is plenty of information now in the scientific literature that would raise a red flag as to the extent of use of glyphosate on everything including your concrete driveway. We've seen that re-evaluation of the safety aspects in a couple of cases put a new light on it. The Indian Supreme Court recently actually insisted on an outside laboratory to do the toxicology analysis for Bt eggplant. The independent laboratory — I believe the one they selected was in New Zealand — stated essentially that the data presented for deregulation of that crop didn't meet international standards for toxicological studies, and that their independent toxicological research found that it wasn't safe for human consumption.

ACRES U.S.A. Despite the difficulty American researchers in particular have experienced, can you now cite much data that wasn't around when GMOs were introduced?

HUBER. There's a fair amount of toxicological data indicating that there are very serious concerns with some of the products. That's also one of the things that has been looked at with infertility and spontaneous abortions. There is an increasing level of glyphosate in our food chain, and with the toxicological data that's now available, the levels are often many times the level that would send up a very serious concern from a clinical laboratory standpoint. Some of that data shows that quite low levels of glyphosate are very toxic to liver cells, kidney cells, testicular cells, and the endocrine hormone system, and it becomes important because all of the systems are interrelated. We're finding fairly significant levels of glyphosate in manure. You have to ask how the chicken got it or how the hog or cattle got it, and of course, that's through their feed. Is it all moving through the animal or is it also into their meat and other tissues? We really don't have a lot of that data. Some of the other countries are collecting it and doing the analysis, and we're just starting to do some in this country. But for the most part it's just been considered so safe that we closed our eyes and said there's no need to do any of that work.

ACRES U.S.A. As you navigate the storm that the untimely release of your letter created, are you finding a certain amount of plain denial of the idea that glyphosate could pose serious problems?

HUBER. I'm finding that a lot of people are really surprised at how many peer-reviewed scientific articles are out there to support what I'm bringing to their attention. Dr. Bill Johnson, a weed scientist at Purdue, documented in a paper he put out last summer that you can't kill a plant with glyphosate in sterile soil, but that it's the soilborne pathogens that are actually the herbicidal mode of action. What you usually hear is that glyphosate inhibits the EPSPS enzyme. Well, just inhibiting the EPSPS enzyme doesn't kill the plant — that's secondary metabolism. When you inhibit that enzyme, you shut down much of the plant's defense mechanisms against these soil-borne fungi. A lot of people aren't aware of the scientific research that's available, and I've had the opportunity to point that out — all the work of Eker, Cakmak, Ozturk, Kremer, Roemheld, Zobiole, etc., are all scientists who have germane concerns which I expressed to the Secretary. Dr. Hannah Mathers at Ohio State shows that glyphosate continues to accumulate in the perennial plant as long as the plant lives. That it continues to accumulate maybe six to eight years, and then finally reaches the level to damage cell walls. One of Dr. Mathers' papers says that this costs Ohio $6.5 million a year in lost ornamental plants through bark-cracking and winter-kill. This kind of environmental stress is because of glyphosate toxicity from the

About Glyphosate

Glyphosate, N-(phosphonomethyl)glycine, is the most extensively used herbicide in the history of agriculture. Weed management programs in glyphosate-resistant (GR) field crops have provided highly effective weed control, simplified management decisions, and given cleaner harvested products. However, this relatively simple, broad-spectrum, systemic herbicide can have extensive unintended effects on nutrient efficiency and disease severity, thereby threatening its agricultural sustainability. A significant increase in disease severity associated with the widespread application of the glyphosate can be the result of direct glyphosate-induced weakening of plant defenses and increased pathogen population and virulence. Indirect effects of glyphosate on disease predisposition result from immobilization of specific micronutrients involved in disease resistance, reduced growth and vigor of the plant from accumulation of glyphosate in meristematic root, shoot, and reproductive tissues, altered physiological efficiency, or modification of the soil microflora affecting the availability of nutrients involved in physiological disease resistance. . . . recommended doses of glyphosate are often many times higher than needed to control weeds . . .

— from Abstract of "Glyphosate Effects on Diseases of Plants"
by G.S. Johal, D.M. Huber, European Journal of Agronomy No. 31 (2009)

weeds that received the glyphosate since it moves out of the weeds' root system and is picked up by the ornamental or the perennial plant. Also, as that weed decomposes, it again releases glyphosate for root uptake into the adjacent plant.

ACRES U.S.A. Are you finding that the actual mechanism of glyphosate is widely misunderstood across the agricultural sector?

HUBER. Right. Most people just accept it as being similar to what we've had with other herbicides, where you have a primary physiological mechanism shutdown so that the chemistry actually does the killing of the plant. With glyphosate, it's only reducing the plant's ability to defend itself from soilborne pathogens. It can stunt the plant for a time before the plant recovers in a sterile soil. But in a non-sterile soil, you shut down that secondary system responsible for defense against those soil pathogens and it's like tying both hands behind the back and letting them trounce on it.

ACRES U.S.A. In your opinion, are the characteristics that led people to regard glyphosate as safer than herbicides of the past the same characteristics that

now make it increasingly troublesome, a threat to the nation's agriculture?

HUBER. Yes, even more so because most of the other herbicides had a full degradation requirement on a time basis. If

INTERVIEW

you had an herbicide that would persist for four or five years, you could only apply that herbicide to a 4th or 5th of the potential acreage. That made sure there was ample time for full biological degradation to occur. With glyphosate we don't necessarily have the degradation. What we have is immobilization. Although there is some degradation that goes on, and that can be demonstrated much better in some soils than in other soils, but it's not a predictable event in many soils. Immobilized glyphosate can be reactivated in soil and be a serious problem for other crops in the rotation. When you realize how little it takes to injure a susceptible crop this is especially important — in one study it only took a 40th of a pound per acre. That's 12 grams or 4/10ths of an ounce spread over an entire acre to prevent 80-90 percent of your root-to-top translocation of the essential nutrients iron, manganese and zinc. Those three very critical micronutrients are going to affect photosynthesis as well as defense reactions and energy reactions in the plant. Glyphosate is a very powerful growth regulator chemical. Even though it can be immobilized readily, it doesn't always stay there.

Monsanto has released a "Statement About Alleged Plant Pathogen Potentially Associated with Roundup Ready Crops." View the contents at *www.monsanto.com/newsviews/Pages/huber-pathogen-roundup-ready-crops.aspx.*

Don Huber, Emeritus Professor, Purdue University, West Lafayette, IN 47907.

REFERENCES

Adams, M., n.d. *Nutrition of the Growing Horse* [online]. Available from: http://www.southernstates.com/articles/nutrition-of-the-growing-horse.aspx [Accessed 10 Nov 2012].

Ahma, J., n.d. *Technical Issues: Oils in the horse diet* [online]. Available from: http://www.athletic-animals.com/oils.htm [Accessed 2 Aug 2012].

Albion Human Nutrition (Ed.). *Why chelated minerals are not created equal* [online]. Clearfield UT. Available from: http://www.albionnutritionalfacts.com/kb/cm-not-equal [Accessed 7 Oct 2012].

Albrecht, W.A., 1975. *Soil Fertility and Animal Health: The Albrecht papers, Vol 2.* edited by Charles Walters. 2nd ed. Kansas City, Mo: Acres U.S.A.

Albright, A. and Stern J.S, 1998. *Adipose Tissue: In: Encyclopedia of Sports Medicine and Science* [online]. Available from: http://www.sportsci.org/encyc/adipose/adipose.html [Accessed 072712].

Alcamo, I.E. and Schweitzer, K., 2001. *CliffsQuickReview biology.* Hoboken, NJ: Wiley Pub.

Alexander, R.M., 1993. The relative merits of foregut and hindgut fermentation. *Journal of Zoology* [online], 231 (3), 391–401. Available from: http://onlinelibrary.wiley.com/store/10.1111/j.1469-7998.1993.tb01927.x/asset/j.1469-7998.1993.tb01927.x.pdf?v=1&t=h2j9u7cj&s=d5ea484a98d900fbe817e7209bb-c8889291bd2b8 [Accessed 22 May 2012].

American Museum of Natural History. *How We Shaped Horses, How Horses Shaped Us* [online]. Available from: http://www.amnh.org/exhibitions/horse/?section=how-shaped&page=howshaped_cii [Accessed 21 Mar 2012].

Andrews, F., *et al.*, 2005. Gastric ulcers in horses. *Journal of Animal Science* [online], Vol. 83 (No. 13), Supplement E18-E21. Available from: http://jas.fass.org/content/83/13_suppl/E18.full [Accessed 04/28/12].

Andrews, M., 2011. *Does restricting grazing really reduce grass intake?* Equine Science Updates [online]. Available from: http://www.equinescienceupdate.com/articles/drgrgi.html [Accessed 4 Apr 2012].

Anna, E., 2008. *About Horse Stables* [online]. Available from: http://www.ehow.com/about_4683966_horse-stables.html [Accessed 18 Mar 2012].

Ashmead, H.D., 2012. *Amino acid chelation in human and animal nutrition.* Boca Raton, FL: Taylor & Francis.

Asplin, K.E., *et al.*, 2007. Induction of laminitis by prolonged hyperinsulinaemia in clinically normal ponies. *The Veterinary Journal* [online], 174 (3), 530–535. Available from: http://www.laminitisresearch.org/downloads/0608/2007_Induction_of_laminitis_by_prolonged_hyperinsulinaemia_in_clinically_normal_ponies_174_530-535.pdf [Accessed 20 Nov 2012].

Astera, M. and Agricola, 2010. *The ideal soil: A handbook for the new agriculture.* St. Cloud MN: Soilminerals.com.

Batmanghelidj, F., 1995. *Your Body's Many Cries for Water: You are not sick, You are thirsty! Don't trust thirst with medications : a preventive and self-education manual for those who prefer to adhere to the logic of the natural and the simple in medicine.* 2nd ed. Falls Church, Va: Global Health Solutions.

Bortoft, H., 1996. *The wholeness of nature: Goethe's way toward a science of conscious participation in nature.* Hudson, NY: Lindisfarne Press.

Bowen, R., 2010. *Microbial Fermentation* [online]. Fort Collins CO. Available from: http://www.vivo.colostate.edu/hbooks/pathphys/digestion/largegut/ferment.html [Accessed 16 May 2012].

Braverman, E.R., 2003. *The healing nutrients within.* 3rd ed. Laguna Beach, CA: Basic Health Publications.

Brownstein, D., 2006. *Salt your way to health.* West Bloomfield, MI: Medical Alternative Press.

Burk, A., 2009. Teaching Basic Equine Nutrition Part II: Equine Digestive Anatomy and Physiology. *University of Maryland Cooperative Extension Fact Sheet* (847b).

Carter, K., 2004. *The history of feeding innovations* [online]. Available from: http://www.horseandhound.co.uk/horsecare/1375/58574.html [Accessed 18 Mar 2012].

Chaffhaye Inc., n.d. [online]. Dell City TX. Available from: http://chaffhaye.com/ [Accessed 18 Mar 2012].

Cichoke, A.J., 1998. *The complete book of enzyme therapy: A complete and up-to-date reference to effective remedies using enzymes, vitamins, and minerals.* Garden City Park, N.Y: Avery Publishing.

Clarkson, N., 2010. *Why did horses die out in North America?* [online]. Available from: http://www.horsetalk.co.nz/features/extinction-176.shtml [Accessed 18 Mar 2012].

Coleman, R., 2001. *Grain Processing: Does it Pay?* [online]. Available from: http://www.ker.com/library/advances/206.pdf [Accessed 10 May 2012].

Eggling, S. and Clackamas Community College, H.B., 2001, 2003. Triesters.

Fletcher, T.M., Janis Christine M., and Rayfield, E.J., 2010. Finite Element Analysis of Ungulate Jaws: Can Mode of Digestive Physiology be Determined? *Palaeontologia Electronica* [online], Vol. 13 (Issue 3). Available from: http://palaeo-electronica.org/2010_3/234/234.pdf [Accessed 19 May 2012].

Frederickson, K. and Noordergraaf, J., 2006. *Equine Gastric Ulcers: Special Care and Nutrition* [online]. North Branch MN. Available from: http://www.sunriseequine.com/Documents/equine_gastric_ulcers.htm [Accessed 04/29/12].

Geor, R.J., 2002. *How Horses Digest Feed* [online]. Lexington KY, American Association of Equine Practitioners. Available from: http://www.aaep.org/health_articles_view.php?print_friendly=true&id=200.

Gill, A., 2009. *Optimizing Bone Formation ... Role of Nutrition, Training and Drug Interaction* [online]. Available from: http://www.amymgillphd.com/library_sub/docs/pdf/Optimizing%20Bone%20Formation-1.pdf [Accessed 27 Sep 2012].

Goodwin, D., 2007. Horse behaviour: evolution, domestication and feralisation. *In:* N. Waran, ed. *The Welfare of Horses.* New York: Springer, 1–18.

Hallebeek, J. and A.C. Beynen, A., 2002. *DIETARY FATS AND LIPID METABOLISM IN RELATION TO EQUINE HEALTH, PERFORMANCE AND DISEASE* [online]. The Netherlands, Department of Nutrition, Faculty of Veterinary Medicine, Utrecht University, The Netherlands. Available from: http://igitur-archive.library.uu.nl/dissertations/2002-0724-153334/c2.pdf [Accessed 29 Jul 2012].

Hanley, T.A., 1982. The Nutritional Basis for Food Selection by Ungulates. *Journal of Range Management* [online], Vol 35 (Issue No 2), 146–151. Available from: http://www.jstor.org/stable/pdfplus/3898379.pdf [Accessed 19 May 2012].

Harvey, S.N., 1987. *Minerals: Right on Target*: Nature's Field.

Hintz, H.F., 2001. *Macrominerals -calcium, phosphorus and magnesium* [online]. Ithaca NY, Cornell University. Available from: http://www.ker.com/library/advances/240.pdf [Accessed 23 Oct 2012].

Hintz, H.F. and Cymbaluk, N.F., 1994. Nutrition of the Horse. *Annual Reviews Nutrition* [online], 14, 243–267. Available from: http://www.annualreviews.org/doi/pdf/10.1146/annurev.nu.14.070194.001331 [Accessed 12 Jun 2012].

Hoffman, R.M., 2003. Carbohydrate Metabolism in Horses. Recent Advances in Equine Nutrition; S.L. Ralston & H.F. Hinds (Eds.). *IVIS*.

Jackson, W.R., 2004. *The Calcium Deception* [online]. Martinez CA, Environmental Health Foundation. Available from: http://ecands.net/pdf/resources/CalcDecptn.pdf [Accessed 18 Sep 2012].

Johnson, E.L. and Duberstein, K.J., 2010. *How to Feed a Horse: Understanding Basic Principles of Horse Nutrition* [online], University of Florida Institute of Food and Agricultural Sciences (IFAS). Available from: http://edis.ifas.ufl.edu/an236 [Accessed 6 Jun 2012].

Jordan, W.J., 2003. *Domestication versus Taming* [online]. Available from: http://circuswatchwa.org/docs/Dr%20W%20Jordan%20Domestication%20versus%20Taming.pdf [Accessed 9 Jun 2012].

Jorgensen, H.-H. and Bosse, A., 2007. *Schüssler tissue salts for horses: Healthy and fit with minerals.* Brunsbek: Cadmos.

Jugdaohsingh, R., 2007. Silicon and bone health. *J Nutr Health Aging*, 11 (2), 99–110.

Kahn, C.M., ed., 2010. *The Merck Veterinary Manual.* Whitehouse Station, NJ: Merck & Co.

Kentucky Equine Research Staff, 1999. *Splittin' hairs: Novel investigations into hair analysis* [online]. Available from: http://www.ker.com/library/equinews/v6n1/v6n114.pdf [Accessed 23 Oct 2012].

Kentucky Equine Research Staff, 2007. Subclinical Acidosis: Is Your Horse At Risk? *EquiNews* [online], 10 (1). Available from: http://www.ker.com/library/equinews/v10n1/v10n106.pdf [Accessed 21 May 2012].

Kentucky Equine Research Staff, 2011a. Fiber: An Important Component in Equine Nutrition. *EquiNews* [online]. Available from: http://equinews.com/article/fiber-an-important-component-in-equine-nutrition [Accessed 31 May 2012].

Kentucky Equine Research Staff, 2011b. Saliva Production and Function in the Horse. *EquiNews* [online]. Available from: http://www.equinews.com/article/saliva-production-and-function-horse [Accessed 3 Apr 2012].

Kentucky Equine Research Staff, 2012. Forage-Only Diet Evaluated for Exercising Horses. *EquiNews* [online]. Available from: http://ker.equinews.com/article/forage-only-diet-evaluated-exercising-horses [Accessed 20 Oct 2012].

Kentucky Performance Products Staff, 2012. *Clarifying Carbohydrates Parts I-III* [online]. Versailles KY, Kentucky Performance Products, LLC. Available from: http://kppusa.com/tips-and-topics/clarifying-carbohydrates-part/ [Accessed 7 Jul 2012].

Kervran, C.L., Rosenauer, H., and Rosenauer, E., 1998. *Biological transmutations.* Woodstock, N.Y: Beekman Publishers.

Kienzle, E. and Zorn, N., 2006. *Bioavailability of Minerals in the Horse - Proceedings of Horse Health Nutrition - Ghent University, 2006* [online]. Ghent University, Merelbeke, Belgium, European Equine Health & Nutrition Congress. Available from: http://www.ivis.org/proceedings/eenhc/2006/kienzle.pdf [Accessed 8 Oct 2012].

King, H.M.e.a. *Shale.* Shale is the most abundant sedimentary rock and is in sedimentary basins worldwide. [online]. Available from: http://geology.com/rocks/shale.shtml [Accessed 7 Oct 2012].

Kohnke, J., 2008. *Understanding Equine Digestion: Some important practical aspects* [online]. Available from: http://www.kohnkesown.com/digestion.pdf [Accessed 17 Apr 2012].

Kopp, K.J., n.d. *Total structural support: a holistic nutritional approach* [online], Arenus. Available from: http://www.arenus.com/Info/Articles/Article/210/total-structural-support-a-holistic-nutritional-approach [Accessed 7 Oct 2012].

Kuhn, T.S., 1970. *The structure of scientific revolutions.* 2nd ed. Chicago: Univ. of Chicago Press.

Laidman, J., 2012. The Secret Life of Fat Suggests New Therapeutic Targets. *Circulation Research* [online], 110, 1049–1051. Available from: http://circres.ahajournals.org/content/110/8/1049.full [Accessed 29 Jul 2012].

Lardy, G. and Poland, C., 2001. *Feeding Management for Horse Owners* [online], North Dakota State University. Available from: http://www.ag.ndsu.edu/pubs/ansci/horse/as953w.htm [Accessed 23 Mar 2012].

Lee, L., Turner, L., and Goldberg, B., 1998. *The enzyme cure: How plant enzymes can help you relieve 36 health problems.* Tiburon, Calif: Future Medicine Pub.

Lemus, R., 2009. *Hay Storage: Dry Matter Losses and Quality Changes* [online]. Mississippi State MS, Mississippi State University Extension Service. Available from: http://msucares.com/pubs/publications/p2540.pdf [Accessed 26 Aug 2012].

Longland, A. and Byrd, B., 2006. Pasture Nonstructural Carbohydrates and Equine Laminitis. *The Journal of Nutrition* [online]. Available from: http://jn.nutrition. org/content/136/7/2099S.full.pdf [Accessed 3 Apr 2012].

Loomis, H.F., 2007. *Enzymes: The key to health*. Madison, WI: 21st Century Nutrition Publishing.

Lowell, B.B. and Flier, J.S., 1997. BROWNADIPOSE TISSUE, b3-ADRENERGIC RECEPTORS, AND OBESITY. *Annual Reviews Medicine* [online], 48, 307–316. Available from: http://www2.uah.es/farmamol/Public/AnnReviews/PDF/Medicine/beta3_adr_obesity.pdf [Accessed 20 Jul 2012].

Macleod, C., 2007. *The truth about feeding your horse*. London: J.A. Allen.

Mende, S.A., n.d. Gastric ulcerations-Mende [online]. Available from: http://wolfecreekequine.drupalgardens.com/sites/wolfecreekequine.drupalgardens.com/files/Gastric%20ulcerations.pdf [Accessed 04/29/12].

Merritt, A.M., 2003a. *Applied Equine Gastrointestinal Physiology* [online]. Gainesville FL. Available from: http://www.as.nchu.edu.tw/lab/211/class/regulatory%20peptides/equine%20GI%20physiology.pdf [Accessed 1 May 2012].

Merritt, A.M., 2003b. *The Equine Stomach: A Personal Perspective (1963-2003)* [online]. Ithaca NY, International Veterinary Information Service (www.ivis.org), 2003. Available from: http://www.ivis.org/proceedings/AAEP/2003/merritt/chapter_frm.asp?LA=1#intragastric [Accessed 04/24/12].

Meunier, C., 2012. *A rising plane of nutrition for the broodmare* [online], Suite101. Available from: http://suite101.com/article/a-rising-plane-of-nutrition-for-the-broodmare-a365198 [Accessed 11 Nov 2012].

Milligan, M., n.d. *What are "colloidal mineral supplements" and where do they come from?* [online]. Salt Lake City UT, Utah Geological Survey. Available from: http://geology.utah.gov/surveynotes/gladasked/gladcoll.htm [Accessed 7 Oct 2012].

National Research Council, ed., 2007. *Nutrient requirements of horses 6th rev. ed.* 6th ed. Washington, D.C: National Academies Press.

Nestle Purina, n.d. *Horses Always Have to Eat* [online]. Available from: http://www.nestlepurina.com/Horses.aspx [Accessed 18 Mar 2012].

New World Encyclopedia contributors, 2008UTC. *Methionine* [online]. Available from: http://www.newworldencyclopedia.org/p/index.php?title=Methionine&oldid=681522 [Accessed 19 Aug 2012UTC].

Ohio State University, n.d. The Horse's Digestive System. *Horse Nutrition*, Bulletin 762-00.

Oke, S. and reviewed by Lawrence, L., 2010. *Vitamins and minerals.* They represent only a tiny portion of your horse's feed intake, but they pack a nutritional wallop [online]. Available from: http://www.thehorse.com/pdf/factsheets/vitamins-minerals/vitamins-minerals.pdf [Accessed 13 Oct 2012].

Olsen, S.L., ed., 2003. *Horses through time.* Niwot, Colo, Oxford: Roberts Rinehart; Oxford Publicity Partnership.

Pagan, J.D., 1998a. *Carbohydrates in Equine Nutrition* [online]. Versailles KY. Available from: http://www.ker.com/library/advances/103.pdf [Accessed 13 May 2012].

Pagan, J.D., 1998b. *Energy and the Performance Horse* [online]. Versailles KY, Kentucky Equine Research Inc. Available from: http://www.ker.com/library/advances/117.pdf [Accessed 5 Aug 2012].

Pagan, J.D., 2009. *Forages: The Foundation for Equine Gastrointestinal Health* [online]. Versailles KY. Available from: http://www.ker.com/library/advances/403.pdf [Accessed 16 May 2012].

Palmer, M., 2008. *Overview of amino acid degradation* [online]. Ontario Canada, University of Waterloo. Available from: http://watcut.uwaterloo.ca/webnotes/Metabolism/page-12.1.html [Accessed 25 Aug 2012].

Rocksandminerals4u.com n.d. *Mineral classification: The dana system* [online] Available from: http://www.rocksandminerals4u.com/mineral_classification.html [Accessed 7 Oct 2012].

Russell, M.A. and Johnson, K.D., 2007. *Selecting Quality Hay for Horses* [online]. West Lafayette IN. Available from: http://www.agry.purdue.edu/ext/forages/publications/ID-190.htm [Accessed 23 May 2012].

Sellnow, L., 2006. Food Factory: Understanding the equine digestive system... *The Horse.com* [online], October, 73–77. Available from: http://www.thehorse.com/pdf/anatomy/anatomy10.pdf [Accessed 23 Mar 2012].

Skipper, L., 2010. *The natural stallion: His behaviour, management and training.* Stockton-on-Tees: Black Tent Publications.

Stewart, C.-B., 2001. *Amino Acid Metabolism Ch 20: Lecture 9: The Urea Cycle (20.3) Breakdown of AAs (20.4) AA Biosynthesis (20.5)* [online]. Available from: http://www.albany.edu/faculty/cs812/bio366/L09_AminoAcidMetab2.pdf [Accessed 19 Aug 2012].

Stover, P.J., 2003. *Fats* [online], Encyclopedia of Food and Culture. Available from: http://www.encyclopedia.com/doc/1G2-3403400217.html [Accessed 29 Jul 2012].

Taiz, L. and Zeiger, E., 2010. *Plant Physiology 5th Ed. Online: Topic 8.14 Fructans.* A companion to Plant Physiology, Fifth Edition [online]. Available from: http://5e. plantphys.net/article.php?ch=t&id=341 [Accessed 10 Jul 2012].

Thiel, R., n.d. *The truth about minerals in nutritional supplements* [online], Doctors' Research. Available from: http://www.doctorsresearch.com/articles3.html [Accessed 7 Oct 2012].

Thomas, H.S., 2012. *Growth Rates in Foals* [online], The Equine Chronicle Online. Available from: http://www.equinechronicle.com/health/growth-rates-in-foals. html [Accessed 11 Nov 2012].

Triforage Horsehae, n.d. [online]. Ontario Canada. Available from: http://triforage. com/ [Accessed 18 Mar 2012].

Triple Crown Nutrition Inc, n.d. [online]. Available from: http://companydatabase. org/c/ship-owners-operators/quality-products/highest-quality/triple-crown-prod-ucts-inc.html [Accessed 13 Jun 2012].

Tuft's Cummings School of Veterinary Medicine, n.d. *How does the horse's stomach work?* [online]. North Grafton MA, Tuft's Cummings School of Veterinary Medicine. Available from: http://vet.tufts.edu/sports/ulcers.html [Accessed 5 Jun 2012].

van den Berg, M., 2011. *Anatomy of the digestive system of the horse: Part 3: Large Intestine* [online]. Available from: https://docs.google.com/view-er?a=v&q=cache:ggt7X_D-VSwJ:www.mberg.com.au/nutrition%2520site/ articles/B%2520Digestive%2520system%2520of%2520the%2520horse%252 0(part%25203).pdf+&hl=en&gl=us&pid=bl&srcid=ADGEESg552yNjJfg2Yb-3zUkzfMRl-B6mJoPIAaFhgPP3czaBrbOOnwu2g3fANzAfGjNH62L-ViI91d-P7aJ7BIBFx83ciw49iwOmb0wmWwuLCpNfZsbLKPUgZ6-FtBrCnCftmioUs Zbbs&sig=AHIEtbQHpP_EcNnjAScl W6bI_umMpBWRbA [Accessed 27 Mar 2012].

Verspoor, R. and Decker, S., 2008. *The dynamic legacy: hahnemann from homeopathy to heilkunst: Book I: An ongoing study of the meaning in the writings of Samuel Hahnemann within the context of the dynamic system of thought.* Manotick ON: Hahnemann Center for Heilkunst.

Wikimedia Foundation Inc, 2012. *Proteinogenic amino acid* [online]. Available from: http://en.wikipedia.org/wiki/Proteinogenic_amino_acid [Accessed 8 Aug 2012].

Wikipedia, 2007. *Compound Feed* [online], Wikimedia Foundation Inc. Available from: http://en.wikipedia.org/wiki/Compound_feed [Accessed 18 Mar 2012].

Wikipedia, 2012. *Equine Anatomy* [online], Wikimedia Foundation Inc. Available from: http://en.wikipedia.org/wiki/Equine_anatomy [Accessed 23 Mar 2012].

Williams, B.A., Verstegen, M.W.A., and Tamminga, S., 2001. Fermentation in the large intestine of single-stomached animals and its relationship to animal health. *Nutrition Research Reviews* [online] (14), 207–227. Available from: http://journals.cambridge.org/download.php?file=%2FNRR%2FNR-R14_02%2FS0954422401000117a.pdf&code=bf80d92204057027d298f403f4d3 8dc7 [Accessed 29 Apr 2012].

Winona State University, 2000. *Introduction to Body Fluids* [online]. Winona MN. Available from: http://www.winona.edu/biology/adam_ip/misc/assignmentfiles/ fluidsandelectrolytes/Introduction_to_Body_Fluids.pdf [Accessed 30 Jun 2012].

Contact Information

Dr. Reagan currently resides on a small farm outside of Knoxville, TN with her family of horses, cats, husband, and mother. She may be contacted through her website or directly via email:

www.horseecology.com
horseecologist@gmail.com